EMERGENCY
Radiation Medical Handbook

The Essential, Mandatory Guide
For Citizens and Responders to Nuclear Events

by
James W. Forsythe M.D., H.M.D.
and
Wayne Rollan Melton

Emergency Radiation Medical Handbook
For Citizens and Responders to Nuclear Events

Century Wellness Publishing
521 Hammill Lane
Reno, NV 895011

Designed by Patty Atcheson-Melton, Wow Design Marketing, Inc.
&
Margie Enlow, NuDirections Graphic Design Marketing

Library of Congress info in publication data

Forsythe, M.D., H.M.D. James W.
Melton, Wayne Rollan

1. Health 2. Environment 3. Nuclear 4. Radiation Sickness

ISBN: 978-0-9848383-2-5

ACKNOWLEDGEMENT

To my entire office staff at Century Wellness Cinic for their encouragement, dedication and loyalty, and all my patients who have suffered from the dangerous effects of radiation.

We want to thank media masters and graphic designers Patty Melton of Wow Design Marketing, and Margie Enlow of NuDirections Graphic Design Marketing for their instant, highly professional quick-turn-around. This book would not have been possible without their leadership, creativity and vision.

Contents

Introduction

Yet, right away people from many geographical areas requesting answers for life-and-death questions that suddenly were posed by the international news media.

The phones at Century Wellness Clinic, my West Coast medical practice, began ringing non-stop in March 2011, within minutes after the nuclear catastrophe erupted in Japan due to a horrific earthquake and tsunami that killed many thousands of people.

"Am I at risk?" people asked, pleading for vital and urgent answers. "What can I do to protect myself and my family from cancer caused by nuclear radiation?"

Just like people from throughout Japan and worldwide, I was caught off guard by the extreme nature of this international emergency.

Yet, right away people from many geographical areas requesting answers for life-and-death questions that suddenly were posed by the international news media.

Before the earthquake and tsunami ignited the horrific nuclear disaster at the Dai-ichi reactors near Fukushima, Japan, people from around the world already were visiting my U.S. medical practice, Century Wellness Clinic for integrative treatments of cancer, pain and other ailments.

11

You should consider this informative handbook an essential tool, a vital guide for use before, during and after radiation emergencies.

I'm one of a handful of integrative medical oncologists in the world. Such professionals practice traditional standard allopathic medical oncology, plus natural treatments such as Homeopathic remedies first developed in Germany, China, and other regions of Asia including Japan.

By March 16, 2011, when foreign countries told their citizens to evacuate Japan as danger from radiation intensified, worried people across the United States and particularly the West Coast began looking to me and other experts for answers.

The level of concern heightened even more after meteorologists announced that radiation from the damaged Japanese nuclear reactors would begin hitting the West Coast of the United States within 10 days—perhaps beginning to peak and surge by March 26 or maybe even sooner.

My Office Staff Went Into Emergency Mode

Determined to meet increasingly strong demand for urgent, sensible information, I immediately directed my office staff to begin assisting me in the development and distribution of this vital "instant book" publication in conjunction with author Wayne Rollan Melton, a former editor-on-loan to "USA Today."

You should consider this informative handbook an essential tool, a vital guide for use before, during and after radiation emergencies. These urgent instances involve the preparation and response to nuclear disasters, plus medical procedures necessary for people exposed to dangerous, potentially life-ending levels of radiation.

Certainly, this publication should be considered as the essential, mandatory handbook for citizens and emergency officials responding to numerous types of radiation tragedies—from severe breakdowns or even meltdowns at nuclear power plants, to survival and response techniques involving weapons of mass destruction such as atomic bombs.

Needless to say, the mainstream news media is crammed with misinformation likely to confuse the general public, possibly leading to ineffective medical treatments. From the start, my objective in producing and distributing this essential handbook remained to set the record straight in regard to radiation sickness.

With these vital factors in mind, you should keep this publication readily available for easy use and reference at all times. In addition, in the wake of the Japan nuclear disaster, many people also are recommending that you distribute additional copies of this publication to your relatives, friends, acquaintances and work associates.

Just as important, preferably well in advance of radiation-related disasters, you should also heed the advice in the pages that follow. Taking the basic and necessary precautions in advance could very

This basic survival and emergency response guide could very well emerge as one of the most essential publications you'll ever read.

well mean the difference between life and death for yourself and for your loved ones.

For best results, you should keep this publication handy in printed form. This essential measure remains vital, largely because in the event of a catastrophic radiation emergency, you likely will lose access to Internet service and even cell phones. When lacking those vital communication tools, having this urgent emergency publication on hand for easy reference could help increase the odds of your potential survival.

This Could be the Most Vital Publication You'll Ever Read

Besides other important reference resources including spiritual publications essential to many religious beliefs, at least from my view as a physician experienced in treating people suffering from radiation exposure, this basic survival and emergency response guide could very well emerge as one of the most essential publications you'll ever read.

Designed as an easy-to-follow, information-packed reference manual, this "Emergency Radiation Medical Handbook" is already emerging as important in today's increasingly complex political and technological environment. Among essential reasons:

- **Terrorists**: While many of us in the Western world remain in denial of this fact, terrorists are busy working non-stop devising ways to inflict weapons of mass destruction on our culture. Many of these weapons involve radiation contamination or nuclear devices as well as chemical and biological weapons.

- **Industry**: Huge multi-national corporations have made monetary profits their top priority, building and operating nuclear power plants described as "harmless" due to so-called fail-safe emergency response systems. Yet, recent history, particularly at the Japanese nuclear power facilities, teaches us that well-intended safety systems can fail and that worst-case scenarios can occur—resulting in widespread death and destruction.

- **Governments**: Recent history also teaches us that even some of the world's most respected democratic governments cannot and should not be trusted in matters involving nuclear tragedies. A prime example of this occurred in Japan during the initial weeks after the disaster, when that nation's government downplayed the severity of the tragedy. As the danger in Japan heightened, even the U.S. government began to realize that many nations public declarations lacked openness and honesty about the urgency of radiation danger.

15

I strongly advise anyone determined to save themselves during a medical emergency involving radiation exposure to learn intricacies of these critical factors, and to take protective measures beforehand.

James W. Forsythe, M.D., H.M.D.

Chapter

1

You Can Expect That Radiation Tragedies Will Occur

For the sake of yourself and for your family, you should assume and be fully aware that horrific radiation-related tragedies will eventually occur in the United States.

Immediatly, you need to understand and fully grasp the fact that I'm not an alarmist. The simple fact of the matter is that our nation's top, most respected Homeland Security officials say the probability of whether we'll ever get attacked by terrorists is not a question of "if" such events will occur—but rather "when" and "how."

To put this into clear, concise and proper perspective, you should think of the 1930s, the decade immediately prior to World War II. At the time, in Germany as the Third Reich solidified and spread its power, many people of the Jewish faith fled Central Europe, immigrating to the United States.

As political tensions surged toward the boiling point and the vilification of Jewish people spread

Most respected Homeland Security officials say the probability of whether we'll ever get attacked by terrorists is not a question of "if" such events will occur—but rather "when" and "how."

17

Those who fled eventually got their well-deserved distinction as forward-thinking and mindfully cautious.

amid the viscious Nazi regime, those who fled the upheaval included the famed genius Albert Einstein.

By some accounts, those who left Europe prior to the war were often considered cowards or at least spineless at the time. But looking back from today's perspective, we know that in the wake of the Holocaust in which millions of Jewish people were slaughtered, those who fled eventually got their well-deserved distinction as forward-thinking and mindfully cautious.

With such events in mind, you should fast-forward to today's complex political and technological environments. The reality of the current situation sends us the clear and undeniable signals that natural environmental, corporate-caused and warfare tragedies involving deadly radiation levels likely will occur.

Why Should Anyone Try to Survive?

From the start, with these clear-cut and undeniable warnings in mind, some people might ask themselves: "If such a tragedy occurs, why would I want to survive anyway? What point would there be to carrying on with life?"

Once again, history can help provide essential and informative answers to such understandable concerns. The region around the 1986 nuclear power plant disaster in the Soviet Union that killed more than 50 people and possibly contaminated nearly 1 million individuals is now surrounded by an expansive populous area.

You can position yourself for potential survival and even prosper after such an event.

And, the United States dropped atomic bombs on the Japan cities of Hiroshima and Nagasaki, killing a combined estimated 150,000 to 246,000 people. Both cities are now thriving communities following extensive rebuilding projects.

While heeding lessons from the past, we know that nuclear catastrophes are survivable, either for those lucky enough to stay out of extreme radiation zones for extensive periods—or for individuals who take vital and urgent precautionary measures such as those techniques described herein.

Indeed, although the imminent threat of nuclear disaster faces us all in the United States, you can and should strive to survive. In all likelihood, by taking the correct precautionary measures, you can position yourself for potential survival and even prosper after such an event.

Follow the Boy Scout Motto ~ "Be Prepared"

Although this might sound trite to some people, the famed motto of the Boy Scouts of America— "Be prepared"—should serve as a clarion call to

What will happen to those who fail to prepare beforehand, for the upcoming radiation events?

every citizen of the United States, as we strive to get ready beforehand for radiation disasters that likely will occur.

While embracing such a strategy, another urgent question comes to mind: "What will happen to those who fail to prepare beforehand, for the upcoming radiation events? What is the most probable outcome for those who intentionally fail to follow these tips?"

Without igniting unnecessary panic, I want you to know that people who fail to follow the simple-to-implement tips in the pages that follow are likely to face:

- **Death**: Those who fail to heed these fairly inexpensive, easy-to-implement tasks in some instances will increase their probability of suffering death from radiation.

- **Financial hardship**: While basic precautionary measures are fairly easy to implement, those who fail to protect their personal resources will have a difficult time financially.

- **Personal loss**: Just as depressing, those who fail to prepare beforehand and to give copies of this publication to their loved ones likely will suffer extensive emotional trauma.

Certainly, the potential losses and personal hardships caused by a massive radiation emergency are extremely difficult to measure. Be that as it may, those who embrace the suggestions within this essential handbook will go a long way toward positioning themselves for a better long-term future.

Certainly, the potential losses and personal hardships caused by a massive radiation emergency are extremely difficult to measure.

This is Far More Serious than the Cold War

Just about anyone in the modern U.S. culture better than 50 years old remembers fallout shelters from the 1950s and 1960s, at the height of the "Cold War" between the United States and the Soviet Union—at the time hailed as the world's two primary international nuclear superpowers.

Looking back, especially because fallout shelters are far less prevalent today in the American culture than during the mid-1900s, those who embraced and followed such emergency preparedness procedures might be perceived as over-reactionary and alarmist. After all, no missiles flew between these nations, and threats between the countries were never openly made—at least in any overt public manner.

By contrast, however, today's current dangers are much more intense and actually "in the works." Our mortal enemies, the terrorists, openly say or indicate that they will attack eventually in a conflagration that some of them describe as a jihad or "holy war." The events of 9-11 gave the

Adding to the distress, some analysts worry about the potential black market sale of components necessary for nuclear bombs.

clear and irrefutable message that these enemies can and will attack suddenly without any regard whatsoever to the sanctity of human life.

Just as disturbing, world events in the past several decades show us that governments and corporations are not forthright about the dangers imposed by nuclear power plants and the resulting dangers of the spread of radiation. Adding to the distress, some analysts worry about the potential black market sale of components necessary for nuclear bombs.

Feeding this proverbial fire even more, huge corporations tell us that nuclear power is extremely safe and that any serious emergencies are unlikely or at least extremely improbable. But, tell that today to anyone who lives in Japan, or the area around Chernobyl in the former Soviet Union, or near Pennsylvania's Three Mile Island Nuclear Generating Station that sustained a partial meltdown in 1979.

Governments Worsen the Safety Problems

The subsequent tips and suggestions further on in this publication are doubly important, when taking into account the fact that all governments are extremely incompetent.

James W. Forsythe, M.D., H.M.D.

Without question, the last thing you should depend on for your survival during a radiation disaster should be any government agency whatsoever. In fact, the world's largest, most powerful or wealthiest nations have failed to protect their citizens from disasters, and those same nations also have failed to adequately respond to widespread emergency conditions once worst-case disaster scenarios erupted.

From the perspective of many observers, our government's emergency response was as slow as a snail.

"The last thing you should depend on for your survival is government," I say, when telling people about the dangers of nuclear radiation. "If you want a guaranteed slow, ineffective and incompetent response, just call your government for help."

As a prime example, consider the tragedy of Hurricane Katrina, which killed at least 1,836 people in and around New Orleans in August 2005. From the perspective of many observers, our government's emergency response was as slow as a snail. In gripping images on live TV broadcast worldwide, hundreds of terrified people were shown clamoring for help at the damaged Superdome in New Orleans.

Worsening matters, some survivors throughout that region began looting stores, also committing murders, thefts and rapes. News reports at the time described snipers, and widespread carnage. The controversy reached a fever pitch due to what some critics hailed as a drastically inadequate government response. Federal Emergency

For another primary example, consider the cases of many thousands—and perhaps tens of thousands—of people who suffered from cancer as a result of above-ground nuclear testing in the Nevada desert in the 1950s and 1960s.

Management Agency Director Michael D. Brown and the superintendent of the New Orleans Police Department, Eddie Compass, resigned amid subsequent investigations.

Never Depend
on the Government

The lessons learned from previous tragedies dictate that you should never depend on, or count on the government to come to your aid during a radiological emergency with any degree of efficiency and dependability.

In fact, history also teaches us that our government is highly insensitive and downright incompetent when factoring in any effort to protect our citizens from nuclear radiation.

For another primary example, consider the cases of many thousands—and perhaps tens of thousands—of people who suffered from cancer as a result of above-ground nuclear testing in the Nevada desert in the 1950s and 1960s. The deadly radioactive fallout from these ill-advised bomb blasts swept into the neighboring states of Utah and Idaho, where many other cancer-related deaths were subsequently reported.

As the many devout readers of my other books already know, particularly "Complete Pain: Forget everything you thought you knew about pain," many movie stars who were on film sets in Utah—downwind of the Nevada explosions—

subsequently died of cancer. The victims included movie stars John Wayne, Dick Powell and Rita Hayworth.

Sadly, our heartless national government did very little if anything to warn people of the urgent need to evacuate from nuclear fallout zones. Lots of us have learned the hard way that our national government is a literal behemoth, moving so slow and so pointlessly that little of any significance gets done with any efficiency in the overall scope of things.

Sadly, our heartless national government did very little if anything to warn people of the urgent need to evacuate from nuclear fallout zones.

A prime example of such governmental ineptitude was exposed by the news media in the wake of initial first-week responses to the Japan disaster. As reported by MSNBC and its news services, some elderly people bore the brunt of the tragedy. Among instances cited in this news story:

- **Abandoned patients**: The report quoted "The Guardian" as stating that a medical staff at a hospital six miles from the damaged Fukushima power plant abandoned 125 elderly Japanese patients, many reported as comatose and "at least 14 subsequently died."

- **Retirement home**: Also as reported by "The Guardian," at least "11 men and women perished inside a retirement home in Kesennuma, where for six days they faced freezing temperatures."

> *"Government is not a solution to our problem— government is the problem."*
>
> -President Ronald Reagan

- **Gymnasium deaths**: The Associated Press described how rescuers moved 14 senior citizens from an evacuation zone near the Fukushima plant to a temporary shelter at a school gym, where they died.

Certainly, as President Ronald Reagan once so eloquently and famously stated, "Government is not a solution to our problem—government is the problem."

Trust Only Yourself, Your Family and Friends Amid a Radiation Emergency

Mindful of the insensitivity of our world's various governments, amid any radiation disaster you should count only on yourself, your family and friends for survival. Any significant aid and assistance that might happen to come from government should be considered as an added blessing.

To be sure, for the most part the people of Japan were let down by their government during the initial weeks after that nation's nuclear power plant disaster. Many of Tokyo's estimated 13 million residents began to flee their country or to move further away from the danger zone during the second week after the tragedy began.

In a culture where respect of country and teamwork are essential, many Japanese citizens spoke openly of their disappointment in their nation's response to the nuclear tragedy.

And, even though that country has perhaps the world's most efficient earthquake preparedness and nationwide emergency response systems, about 10 days after the tragedy some people in the tsunami zone started complaining that "our country is failing us. They're leaving us to die."

Television news viewers from other nations watched, dumbstruck as people staying in makeshift community shelters in destruction zones began running out of food, and while supplies of essential clean water decreased to drastically low levels.

Sadly, once again, those events served as another reminder of how national governments consistently fail to adequately serve the very people that they're dedicated to protect. Certainly, I'll be the target of much criticism for even pointing this out. Even so, anyone determined to pursue survival should carefully take such factors into consideration.

Sadly, once again, those events served as another reminder of how national governments consistently fail to adequately serve the very people that they're dedicated to protect.

My staff worked around-the-clock, non-stop in a focused effort to get these vital details into your hands as soon as possible after the Japan tragedy began.

Time is of the Essence When Learning These Skills

With all these urgent factors in mind, time is of the essence for any person determined to learn radiation survival skills and to implement these measures before such tragedy strikes.

Determined to satisfy the public's vital need for this essential information, my staff worked around-the-clock, non-stop in a focused effort to get these vital details into your hands as soon as possible after the Japan tragedy began.

As you might imagine, from the very start this self-imposed task seemed formidable, since at the time in Japan many tens of thousands or perhaps even millions of people faced potential contamination from radiation almost from the very start.

Certainly, as you'll soon discover, this essential handbook deals with far more than Japan's tragic nuclear situation because similar events remain possible worldwide.

"People have a right to know about the seriousness of the dangers that they face," I told key members of my communications team. "We need to teach people the best, most effective methods of protecting themselves and their families—plus where and how to seek vital medical treatments if and when they suspect they have been exposed to radiation."

Meantime, my extensive background in treatments of cancers and in military situations motivated me to assume an essential and much-needed leadership role in this regard. A Vietnam War veteran and a retired Nevada Army National Guard colonel, I'm the author of many books—including one book co-written by best-selling author Suzanne Somers, a popular TV star and media personality.

Experience Motivated Me to Set the Facts Straight

Now entering my fifth decade as a practicing medical oncologist, I have treated many thousands of patients including streams of people who eventually died of cancer caused by above-ground nuclear bomb tests conducted in the Nevada desert in the 1950s and early 1960s.

Sadly, many of the people exposed to those radiation episodes are just now beginning to present or show cancer symptoms caused by these incidents from many decades ago.

As you might imagine, largely as a result of my medical clinic's proximity to these former nuclear test sites, I have treated countless cases of thyroid cancer, which, if untreated, can be fatal. This cancer is perhaps the most prevalent ailment suffered by people exposed to radiation.

I have treated many thousands of patients including streams of people who eventually died of cancer caused by above-ground nuclear bomb tests conducted in the Nevada desert in the 1950s and early 1960s.

An increasingly large percentage of my cancer patients regained good and vibrant health— many after formerly being at "death's doorstep."

And, like a vast majority of other traditional standard medical oncologists during the 1970s and 1980s, a vast majority of my Stage IV cancer patients from that era died as a result of the disease. Extreme nausea and pain caused by traditional chemotherapy often compounded their suffering during the final stages of their lives.

Determined to find a better, more effective way to treat cancer patients, during the mid-1990s I also became a certified, licensed and practicing homeopath. While often shunned by so-called traditional doctors, homeopathy is sometimes hailed as an "alternative medicine" outside the mainstream of traditional diagnosis and treatments.

While my decision to add homeopathy to my services sparked the ire of many so-called traditional doctors, the results of this career transition became irrefutable. You see, until adding homeopathy to my repertoire, the vast majority of my results mirrored those of most other traditional medical oncologists—almost all my Stage IV cancer patients died.

The results made a dramatic change for the better when I incorporated homeopathy into my medical practice. An increasingly large percentage of my cancer patients regained good and vibrant health— many after formerly being at "death's doorstep."

James W. Forsythe, M.D., H.M.D.

Combining Eastern and Western Medicines Beats Cancer

As growing numbers of people from Asia and across the Western United States face the potential dangers of radiation exposure, I'm one of a few integrative medical oncologsts who have experience in some degree of success in treating cancer patients who have:

- **Nuclear Contamination**: Patients who acquired cancer as a direct result of their personal exposure to radiation from nuclear fallout.

- **Integrative Treatments**: Received combinations of traditional and non-traditional medicines or treatments, in many cases enabling patients to bounce back to good health.

Sparking the ire and criticism of many so-called traditional medical oncologists, I'm also quick to point out that the traditional cancer chemotherapy treatments most often employed by such medical practitioners often generate more harm than good among patients.

"At the start of this international medical emergency, we need to take a strong stand in this regard," I told my communications staff as the Japan radiation emergency intensified. "Standard medical oncologists will not like what I'm going

Conventional medical oncologists will not like what I'm going to tell the world.

Just because someone has a medical degree or is a scientist, are they qualified to tell millions of worried people how to respond to this situation?

to tell the world. But consumers everywhere have a right to know the truth. To give them any other details to the contrary would be deceitful and disrespectful to the general public."

My Level of Concern Increased

Just as the initial work began for the publication you're reading now, my level of personal concern began to intensify.

You see, the problem became exacerbated from a public relations standpoint, when TV journalists and radio shows began interviewing so-called experts analyzing the Japanese nuclear reactor tragedy. The paradoxical situation made me wonder, "Just because someone has a medical degree or is a scientist, are they qualified to tell millions of worried people how to respond to this situation?"

Without mentioning specific names here, suffice it to say that many of these so-called experts were identified as the head of "such-and-such" a university's research department or standard in-house science experts employed by TV networks.

Yet, what real-world experience did these specific individuals have at treating radiation-caused cancers? Have any of these professionals successfully treated such ailments on a massive scale? And, with just as much urgency, why should we believe what they say?

While taking those interviews to heart, imagine how I felt upon hearing such statements, when considering the fact that I'm among only a handful of medical professionals worldwide with such essential qualifications and experience.

To help put this in perspective, imagine yourself in my shoes. What if you were one of the few doctors in the world with first-hand, extensive experience on how to save the lives of many individuals—perhaps millions of them—from the ravages of a horrific disaster? For most people, I suppose, I imagine the answer would be: "I would do everything possible to get the word out, to give specific, urgent, vital and easy-to-understand details in a manner that enables the public to take immediate, positive action."

Thank God those of us in the Western culture live in a society where free speech enables us to get the word out, creating a communications pathway for medical professionals to set the record straight.

The News Media is Like an Errant Fire Hose

Thank God those of us in the Western culture live in a society where free speech enables us to get the word out, creating a communications pathway for medical professionals to set the record straight.

This saving grace became more evident than ever during the first week following the onset of the international Japan nuclear power tragedy. While at home flipping through the various TV news channels as that tragic event unfolded, most major

Even so, at least from my personal view, some networks seemed to give incomplete or confusing information on everything from health dangers to evacuation methods.

broadcasts showed the same magnetic, compelling and unforgettable images of the earthquake, tsunami and the disabled nuclear power reactors.

Even so, at least from my personal view, some networks seemed to give incomplete or confusing information on everything from health dangers to evacuation methods.

Herein rests the key, essential objectives of this publication, "Emergency Radiation Medical Handbook." In the pages that follow you will discover:

- **Avoidance**: Methods of avoiding contamination or at least decreasing the probability of such an occurrence.

- **Cancer types**: The most prevalent types of cancers suffered by those exposed to dangerously high levels of nuclear contamination.

- **Treatment methods**: The essential methods of treating specific types of cancer likely to be suffered by such individuals.

- **Foods and beverages**: The various foods and beverages likely to generate serious levels of radiation, before passing this dangerous substance on to people.

- **Radioactive Elements**: The specific elements generated by radiation, plus the certain types of cancers or ailments that each is likely to generate.

- **Generational problems**: Specific ailments or symptoms suffered by people exposed to radiation, negative or detrimental characteristics likely to be passed on to subsequent generations.

- **Prevention methods**: How can society prevent or lessen the likelihood of similar catastrophic events?

With the extreme potential dangers of the recent tragedy in mind, you should consider this as the required "Emergency Handbook," essential for all consumers, medical professionals and first-response rescue personnel.

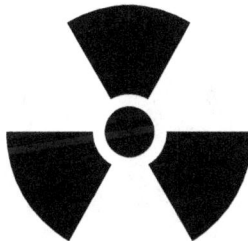

With the extreme potential dangers of the recent tragedy in mind, you should consider this as the required "Emergency Handbook," essential for all consumers, medical professionals and first-response rescue personnel.

35

Chapter

2

Serious Nuclear Power Plant Accidents are Fairly Common

Despite the nonsense and propaganda spewed by our government, politicians and high-paid lobbyists employed by the electric power industry, nuclear accidents are fairly common worldwide. This is the conclusion that was reached in a 2010 publication by Benjamin K. Sovacool, "A Critical Evaluation of Nuclear Power and Renewable Electricity in Asia."

If these reports are true, as some analysts apparently fear, a disturbingly high total of 56 of the 99 accidents occurred at nuclear power plants in the United States.

Sovacool's report gives us the critical and urgent news that there have been 99 accidents at nuclear power plants worldwide since the 1986 Chernobyl disaster. If these reports are true, as some analysts apparently fear, a disturbingly high total of 56 of the 99 accidents occurred at nuclear power plants in the United States.

Word of Sovacool's discoveries might come as shocking and highly disturbing news, especially to many U.S. citizens who heard nothing but rosy, highly positive reports about the American nuclear

As if seizing the opportunity to jump into the worldwide media spotlight, lots of these elected leaders openly embraced what they described as the safe and essential nuclear power industry.

power industry during coverage of the 2011 Japan tragedy.

Imagine the shock and disgust many observers who knew of these truths must have felt, when high-paid public relations officials for the nuclear power industry were interviewed on nationwide TV. One by one, these spokespeople told what they described as a highly safe industry where the potential for horrible disasters was said to be "almost impossible."

Puppets or marionettes controlled by their high-power, big-money donors, many top politicians also got into the act. As if seizing the opportunity to jump into the worldwide media spotlight, lots of these elected leaders openly embraced what they described as the safe and essential nuclear power industry.

But if these facilities actually are as safe as officials claim, then why did they fail to mention the many nationwide nuclear disasters chronicled by Sovacool? And, why did the news media for the most part fail to ask our elected officials and the nuclear power industry personnel to give reasons for the many nuclear disasters?

The Secret Numbers about Accidents Are Disturbing

With little doubt, those who run and embrace the U.S. nuclear power industry will throw a fit, once they learn that this vital and essential Emergency Radiation Handbook gives some of the basics on their industry's many failures.

More important, what does all this ultimately mean for you and for your family?

Well, from my perspective, there can be little denying that much of the American public faces severe danger from a future potential radiation disaster sparked by the nuclear power industry. As if to emphasize or at least to admit the danger, the International Atomic Energy Agency has made the noble decision to list at least 23 of these incidents on its official Website, IAEA.org.

Straight in the face of such disturbing information, our politicians have failed us, particularly by refusing to ask for more answers and for in-depth investigations of the U.S. nuclear power industry—especially in the wake of the Japan disaster. Meantime, although President Barack Obama promised that all nuclear reactors in the U.S. would undergo review, from my view the public should remain skeptical—particularly in the wake of our government's dismal track record.

To their credit, fresh on the heels of the Japan tragedy as the dangers heightened in that Asian nation, officials in Germany announced their government's plan to take a "measured exit" from nuclear power. Seizing a courageous stand that many nuclear power industry officials likely despised, German Chancellor Angela Merkel

The United States has
a total of 104 operational nuclear power plants, with one additional facility under construction.

made a bold and fresh statement to her nation's parliament.

"When the apparently impossible happens in a highly developed country such as Japan, then the whole situation changes," Merkel said. In the face of criticism from some business sectors, Merkel took the courageous stand of shutting down seven of Germany's oldest nuclear power plants for inspection.

"We will use the moratorium period, which we deliberately set to be short and ambitious, to drive the change in energy policy and accelerate it wherever possible, as we want to reach the age of renewable energy as quickly as possible," Merkel said.

Our Nuclear Power Industry Remains Huge

The United States has a total of 104 operational nuclear power plants, with one additional facility under construction. An additional nine similar facilities are in the planning stages, and another 22 are in the proposal stage, according to a June 2009 publication by the U.S. Energy Information Administration.

The same organization estimates that the existing operational facilities generate nearly 20 percent of the electrical power currently consumed in the United States.

Needless to say, with so much money involved, are the officials who approve, regulate and operate these facilities putting you and your family at excessive risk?

This seems a reasonable question to ask when taking into consideration the fact that all of the currently operating nuclear power plants in the United States are at least 37 years old. By almost every account, the expansion of the U.S. nuclear power industry seems to be easing along at a slower pace.

Meantime, the aging infrastructure of the U.S. nuclear power industry might begin to show signs of aging. Even old cars and reusable NASA space shuttles have required continual upgrading, rebuilding and extensive maintenance that included sporadic but necessary shutdowns for essential refurbishing work.

Worries Intensified Across the United States

Amid rising public concern in the wake of the Japan earthquake and tsunami, observers worried about the danger to the 23 stressed nuclear power plants in the U.S. which are in similar design to the nuclear power facilities in Asia. Worsening matters, the only two nuclear power plants on the U.S. West coast on the edge of the Pacific Ocean

Officials insisted that each Golden State facility was built to withstand a tsunami of at least 25 feet, while also capable of withstanding temblors ranging from magnitudes of 7.0 to 7.5 on the Richter Scale.

were designed to withstand tsunamis and temblors far less severe than the catastrophic events that rocked the Land of the Rising Sun.

Critics seized upon the controversy, calling for inspections by federal regulators at the California plants at San Clemente and at Diablo Canyon.

Officials insisted that each Golden State facility was built to withstand a tsunami of at least 25 feet, while also capable of withstanding temblors ranging from magnitudes of 7.0 to 7.5 on the Richter Scale.

By comparison, the Japan earthquake which initially killed an estimated total of more than 10,000 people before death tolls mounted further, reached a magnitude of 9.0. According to CBS News, the Japan tsunami reached 76 feet high. That's more than three times larger than the Golden State facilities were built to withstand.

"Across the board, the NRC (Nuclear Regulatory Commission) has not set standards at a high enough level to protect the public from accidents that are more credible and plausible than previously considered," Ed Lyman of the watchdog group Union of Concerned Scientists said at a Washington, D.C., press conference as the Japan tragedy intensified.

Amid the resulting public uproar, the news media reported that in 2008 a California Energy Commission report stated that there were no safeguards at the San Onofre Nuclear Generating Station for withstanding an earthquake of a magnitude exceeding 7.0. Officials noted that when the plant was built in the 1960s that was the level that designers had expected.

Some Officials Recognized the Potential Danger

To their credit, at least some regulatory officials recognized and acknowledged the report's findings, ordering a new earthquake and tsunami risk analysis at the San Onofre facility— mandating that its operators use the latest technology while seeking renewal of the plant's operating license set to expire in 2022, according to the "San Diego Tribune."

Amid heightened concerns during the initial month after the Japan reactor disaster, The "Los Angeles Times" reported on March 31, 2011, that the San Onofre plant's operators proposed a multimillion-dollar study that "would use new technology to better assess seismic conditions near the northern San Diego County complex."

News of the proposed investigation came one day after lawyers for a "former manager at San Onofre announced they had filed a lawsuit against the company, saying the man was fired after he raised other employees' safety concerns with the Nuclear Regulatory Commission,"The Times" said.

On the downside, however, while the bureaucratic wheels spin over a period of many years and even decades, much of the general public still faces potential danger from such facilities.

Of course, once again it's important to stress that history tells us that scientists sometimes proclaim vastly differing opinions or theories.

On the downside, however, while the bureaucratic wheels spin over a period of many years and even decades, much of the general public still faces potential danger from such facilities.

Discovery News reported that although the California Edison utility gave its initial submission of the required report on the Diablo Canyon facility to the Public Utilities Commission, the document "lacked a three-dimensional seismic analysis that the agencies requested."

For average citizens across California and particularly within the potential downwind zone of catastrophic incidents at the Japan nuclear reactors, the utility's apparent lack of an adequate response serves as yet another reminder that we all need to remain vigilant. Yes, as individuals and families, we cannot and should not depend on government and particularly on huge corporations to ensure our physical safety.

From the view of University of California at Berkeley seismologist Peggy Hellweg, as quoted by Discovery News, the probability of a tsunami hitting either or both of the Southern California facilities on the Pacific shore is unlikely because the Golden State's coast is not as exposed as the shore areas of Japan. Hellweg also doubts that earthquake faults off the Southern California coast could generate temblors with the power of the Japan quake.

"The size of the earthquake depends on the size of the uninterrupted fault you have," Hellweg told Discovery News. "The length of those faults (off the Golden State coast) isn't long enough to get a magnitude 8 or 9."

Of course, once again it's important to stress that history tells us that scientists sometimes proclaim vastly differing opinions or theories. When nuclear safety is involved, officials in Japan miscalculated—they were flat-out wrong when predicting what they considered the worst-case potential disasters there. So, for now, a looming question remains for us in the United States: "Is there a possibility our scientists are making a similar mistake?"

At this rate, if the industry's growth holds steady as these corporate officials predict, such facilities will scatter across many nations worldwide.

The Nuclear Power Industry is Spreading Fast

Like a slap in the face of the entire world, the nuclear power industry keeps charging full steam ahead amid ongoing and relentless efforts to expand their industry.

Disturbingly and despite the lessons we should have learned from previous disasters at such facilities, by 2015 at least one new nuclear power facility will open somewhere in the world every five days. Those are the estimates of the World Nuclear Association, as described in "Plans for New Reactors Worldwide."

Once again, sadly, we have a situation where you'll be forced to fend for yourself in order to survive physically, financially, and even mentally.

At this rate, if the industry's growth holds steady as these corporate officials predict, such facilities will scatter across many nations worldwide. Imagine the dangers involved as numerous countries and diverse cultures strive to end their reliance on increasingly expensive fossil fuels and to eliminate extensive metal emissions that also cause health hazards.

Ultimately, while the danger for irreversible human error persists at nuclear power plants, people facing the worst dangers will be those in the most concentrated regions of the world's burgeoning population that is rapidly approaching 7 billion souls.

Of course, with all these many interlinked factors involved, no one can say with 100 percent certainty that a nuclear power plant accident of major import will occur within the United States in the near future. Yet, as the infrastructure of those existing facilities continues to age, the increasingly intense possibility of a new disaster looms.

Our Country Lacks Strong Leadership on Energy

As you continue to learn the essential radiation disaster survival basics, keep in mind that our country lacks the strong, vibrant and decisive leadership necessary to end our reliance on fossil fuels and on nuclear energy. For the most part, any effort to revert to clean "renewable energies" such as wind power and solar energy have been weak, indecisive and lacking vibrant focus—at least when considered on a massive scale.

But what do these oversights mean for you and for your family?

Once again, sadly, we have a situation where you'll be forced to fend for yourself in order to survive physically, financially, and even mentally. After all, everyday folks already have enough to worry about in today's fast-paced, hectic and confusing society without having to devote a majority of their time and personal energies on such issues.

Nonetheless, due to the increasing intensity of these societal problems, you are now finding yourself faced with no other option than to learn the basic survival techniques and how to minimize potential damage to your own personal and financial well being.

Since an estimated 2,982 people died in the jetliner tragedies of September 11, 2001, the number of successful terrorist attacks has swelled worldwide.

The Terrorist Problem Multiplies the Danger Multi-Fold

As if the nuclear power industry's nagging problems weren't already enough to give us a non-stop migraine, the imminent and almost-certain threat imposed by terrorists forces peace-lovers everywhere to take decisive measures for protecting themselves.

Emergency Radiation

Those specializing in these tactics want to kill people by the tens of thousands or even millions on a massive scale, through the use of nuclear weapons and radiological devices.

Since an estimated 2,982 people died in the jetliner tragedies of September 11, 2001, the number of successful terrorist attacks has swelled worldwide. And, although authorities have managed to thwart a wide range of planned wide-scale attacks since then, many analysts tell us that it's just a matter of time before another massive incident succeeds.

"We're in a new world," Condoleezza Rice, former U.S. Secretary of State, has been quoted as saying. "We're in a world where the possibility of terrorism married up with technology, could make us very, very sorry that we didn't act."

In a way, terrorists are like radiation at least in the sense that we rarely see or recognize them with the naked eye until it's far too late to take immediate and decisive action. The danger of potential radiation contamination comes into play when such selfish attackers seek to engage in what military analysts label "environmental terrorism."

Terrorists focused on these tactics target a city, state or region's natural resources, everything from crops and water supplies to corporate infrastructures such as nuclear power plants. Yes, here again comes a reminder that those who intend to inflict extreme harm on the United States continue to work non-stop to carry out their objective.

Any worries of a wide-scale attack intensify when recognizing the irrefutable fact that these enemies of the United States and other nations seek to engage in what military analysts call "nuclear terrorism." Those specializing in these tactics want to kill people by the tens of thousands or even millions on a massive scale, through the use of nuclear weapons and radiological devices.

Such radiological weapons are designed to spread massive amounts of deadly radioactive materials, usually via the use of standard or conventional explosives.

These strategies include the planning and implementation of attacks on facilities that contain devices that involve massive amounts of deadly radiation. Cognizant of the increasingly intense need to address this issue, in 2005 the United Nations held what authorities hailed as the "International Convention for the Suppression of Acts of Nuclear Terrorism."

Among key potential targets the officials identified were nuclear power plants and nuclear reactors. With just as much urgency, international leaders actively sought to impose stringent reporting procedures via the International Atomic Energy Agency.

Disturbingly, international police investigators have identified increasingly dangerous potential weapons labeled as "suitcase nukes." These devices supposedly are so portable that they actually could be delivered in a suitcase, although some observers openly complain that any reports of such devices are unverifiable.

Yet, as you learn more about how to protect yourself from the potential ravages of radiation, always remain aware that various other radiological weapons either exist or are possibly in the development stage as terrorists plan their attacks.

Described as "miniaturized nuclear weapons," such small-scale weapons of mass destruction supposedly could cause death on a massive scale.

While some analysts doubt the existence of these devices, at least judging by a wide variety of published accounts, there seems to be widespread agreement on the dangers of "dirty bombs." Such radiological weapons are designed to spread massive amounts of deadly radioactive materials, usually via the use of standard or conventional explosives.

The explosion of a dirty bomb could cause immediate deaths or injury, while victims who come in contact with radiation face the short- or long-term possibility of severe illnesses including cancer. But analysts question whether dirty bombs would contain enough radiation to inflict such maladies or even deaths.

Putting worries somewhat at ease, the U.S. Department of Energy has concluded that radiation exposure would be "fairly high but not fatal" for anyone who stays for one year in a dirty bomb's destruction zone that was never cleaned to remove radiation contamination.

Call Them "Weapons of Mass Hysteria"

While dirty bombs are likely to inflict deaths on a massive, widespread scale, some analysts hail such devices as "weapons of mass hysteria" due to the widespread fear and panic such explosions are likely to cause.

Yet, as you learn more about how to protect yourself from the potential ravages of radiation, always remain aware that various other radiological weapons either exist or are possibly in the development stage as terrorists plan their attacks. Among known devices or delivery systems:

- **Radiological warfare**: Terrorists or combatants surreptitiously introduce extremely harmful levels of radiation into the basic and necessary supply systems upon which human life depends. These infrastructures include the food supply chain, plus local, county and municipal water delivery systems. From the terrorist point of view, hopefully the intended victims will not notice the extreme danger until after they have been fatally contaminated with extremely high levels of radioactive materials.

- **Salted bombs**: Although not technically nuclear bombs, these devices are intended to rapidly spread fatal levels of radioactive fallout. When deployed properly from the terrorist's perspective, these explosions render expansive areas of land—perhaps

From the terrorist point of view, hopefully the intended victims will not notice the extreme danger until after they have been fatally contaminated with extremely high levels of radioactive materials.

Such retooling of standard, high-power weaponry could very well generate what I personally consider cataclysmic materials.

entire cities, towns and communities—virtually uninhabitable. In the process, the terrorist would strive to immediately kill as many people as possible, while inflicting fatal levels of radioactive materials on any individuals who survive the initial explosions. According to a 2002 publication, "Nuclear, Biological and Chemical Warfare," a Hungarian-American physicist, Leo Szilard, introduced the concept of salted bombs in 1950 in an effort to show that weapons technology could progress to where combatants could effectively end human life on earth. The same publication also states that salted bombs are designed to increase the production of radioactive fallout via the weapon-based delivery of certain elements—in an effort generate radioactive isotopes.

By some accounts, certain weapons of mass destruction such as hydrogen bombs can be converted into salted bombs. Such retooling of standard, high-power weaponry could very well generate what I personally consider cataclysmic materials. While the bombardment effect of such a device might be somewhat curtailed in the retooling process, the overall extreme danger from radiation within blast zones could continue for extended periods.

As a physician fully dedicated to treating and eradicating cancers of many kinds, I feel motivated to give you the vital, urgent and compelling news that such weaponry could cause the extensive widespread loss of life. With this fully understood, as citizens possessing personal rights and responsibilities, we Americans collectively have a moral obligation to do whatever we can to take decisive, legal measures to protect ourselves from such outcomes.

Expect Terrorists to Employ Additional Evil Tactics

With just as much viciousness and heartless demeanor, terrorists also are likely to plan other types of attacks designed to generate the widespread dissemination of extremely dangerous radioactivity. Among the worst, most violent potential tactics:

- **Nuclear weapons**: Either acquire nuclear bombs on the black market, or amass the specific, hard-to-obtain materials necessary to build such devices. Some national security agencies such as the Central Intelligence Agency reportedly worry that terrorists or other national enemies might be busy striving to make such acquisitions.

- **Nuclear Reactors**: Instigate sudden, extreme attacks on nuclear power plants, overtaking the facilities before possibly blowing them up or destroying them in other ways—in order to spread

Meantime, no strong, extreme protective procedures appear in place at such facilities at least as far as any military presence or extensive policing infrastructures.

53

extremely harmful levels of radiation over widespread areas. Amid news coverage on the Japan tragedy, officials or spokesmen at various U.S. nuclear power plants stressed that they had anti-terrorist mechanisms in place. Yet, for the most part it seems authorities remain mum on specific details of such protective measures. Meantime, no strong, extreme protective procedures appear in place at such facilities at least as far as any military presence or extensive policing of infrastructures. Certainly a handful of security guards each holding a holstered revolver would be no match for a well-honed, highly trained team of terrorist commandos.

- **Sudden attacks**: Some counter-terrorism experts also have chronicled their persistent, non-stop worries that terrorists will try to take over nuclear submarines, hijack jetliners with the intention of ramming them into nuclear power plants, or even swarm onto our domestic U.S. military bases in an effort to abscond with or deploy nuclear weapons from the nation's existing weapons stockpiles.

- **Smuggling**: Terrorists and perhaps standard-enemy nations might strive to sneak weapons of unthinkable power into the United States, with the express purpose of attacking innocent Americans on their own soil. This undoubtedly hails as one of the biggest worries of our national security experts, particularly since just one standard nuclear bomb could potentially cause far more immediate deaths and long-term radioactive damage than many of the less powerful weapons combined.

"To penetrate and dissipate the clouds of darkness, the general mind must be strengthened by education."

-Benjamin Franklin

"Avoid popularity if you would have peace," advised Abraham Lincoln, the legendary and iconic 16th president of the United States. These concise and vibrant words of wisdom from more than 150 years ago still ring true today, as our nation's leaders strive to make tough and increasingly difficult decisions in efforts to keep the USA safe.

Eager to fully embrace and covet such focused determination, each of us needs to do his or her part to educate ourselves on the best and most effective methods to survive such potential radiological attacks. Indeed, as founding father Benjamin Franklin once proclaimed, "To penetrate and dissipate the clouds of darkness, the general mind must be strengthened by education." Seizing the proverbial torch of freedom in this regard, let us move forward together in succeeding to survive from the forces of nature and from the efforts of any enemy who might strive to cause us serious harm.

Put into the hands of Islamic extremists, such weaponry certainly could wreak massive, widespread destruction on the United States if deployed effectively and without warning.

America's Allies Also are Targets of Radiological Weaponry

Heightening international concerns, many of the USA's most strident and loyal allies of longtime good standing also have been targeted by terrorists for mass destruction.

In 2006, "The Guardian" quoted the Foreign Affairs office in Great Britain as stating that intelligence officials gained information leading them to believe an attack on their nation by the al-Qaida terrorist organization was being planned. During that period and numerous times since then, allied governmental intelligence experts have reported discovering "lots of chatter" on terrorist Websites about probable or planned attacks.

Putting concern levels to a fever pitch, numerous news accounts have described various incidents where terrorists attacked three nuclear power plants in Pakistan. Did these incidents stem from possible attempts to gain access to that nation's nuclear arsenal? And, if so, would the assailants have strived to use those weapons on the United States?

Varying news reports have indicated that U.S. security officials have declined to discuss whether such efforts may have been a possibility. Whatever the case, unconfirmed and apparently unverifiable reports spread that Pakistan possesses up to 80 nuclear warheads. Put into the hands of Islamic extremists, such weaponry certainly could wreak massive, widespread destruction on the United States if deployed effectively and without warning.

According to CNN, sometimes known as the Cable News Network, author and nuclear weapons expert David Wright has stated his concerns that in the wake of many leaks of classified information in Pakistan that "you have to worry that it (nuclear weapons) could be acquired" there.

Buoyed by the knowledge of such increasingly dangerous situations, while careful to avoid panic you should strive to make preparations for what many international terrorism experts seem to fear will be imminent, widespread attacks on the United States.

Focused and determined to wrap a tight noose around this potential problem, in 2002 the United States generated an international effort to cut the probability that terrorists or other enemies would successfully obtain uranium.

Soviet Challenges Likely Exacerbated the Nuclear Problems

Worsening matters on a widespread international scale, America's national security experts have expressed concerns that terrorists might seek to purchase or obtain enriched uranium crucial in the construction of nuclear bombs.

Focused and determined to wrap a tight noose around this potential problem, in 2002 the United States generated an international effort to cut the probability that terrorists or other enemies would successfully obtain uranium. Authorities aimed the

For the first 60 years, the clock's time had been set to indicate how close the planet was to global nuclear war, an international holocaust that likely represents the annihilation of the human race.

bulk of these efforts in 16 countries at 24 Soviet-style nuclear power facilities.

For those of us cognizant enough to pay close attention to the scattered, sporadic and hodgepodge-style news reports of such occurrences, the news should inspire increased personal efforts to take decisive action for self-preservation.

An ancient Latin poem by Horace, a Roman from the first century before Christ, urges that we "seize the day (or 'carpe diem,' the Latin term)—putting as little trust as possible in the future." Certainly the continual and disturbing influx of information about what many of us perceive as the likely coming radiological attacks serves as an unavoidable wake-up call.

After all, judging by streams of verifiable news accounts on this vital and urgent topic, the dangers facing those of us in the United States are more severe than ever—perhaps even more so than during the height of the cold war.

Always Pay Close Attention to these Mounting Dangers

To put this into clear and concise perspective, always keep the following vital information at the forefront of your mind. Since 1947, the "Bulletin of Atomic Scientists" has maintained what they appropriately call "the Doomsday Clock."

Now entering the third human generation since this interesting and compelling system began, the clock is used as a signal on how close mankind is to the scientists' estimate of global disaster. These experts tell us that the closer to midnight that they put the clock, the closer the world is to such a catastrophic and cataclysmic event.

For the first 60 years, the clock's time had been set to indicate how close the planet was to global nuclear war, an international holocaust that likely represents the annihilation of the human race. Under such a scenario, much of the world or the entire planet would become uninhabitable due to widespread catastrophic nuclear bomb detonations. Since 2007, besides global nuclear war the clock also has factored in the technologies that change the global weather climate, plus the dangers imposed by nanotechnology—the intentional manipulation of matter. Along with nuclear bombs, scientists worry that climate changes and nanotechnology could play essential roles in the destruction of mankind.

During that period, they set the clock back to 17 minutes before midnight in the wake of the Strategic Arms Reduction Treaty between the United States and the Soviet Union.

In recent years, the scientists have set the clock at just six minutes before midnight, the so-called "doomsday hour." Officials had initially set the clock at just seven minutes to midnight when the timekeeper first went into operation just a few years after the end of World War II.

Since then, scientists have reset the clock at least 17 times, in each instance rewound in accordance

In January 2010 when scientists set the time back by just one minute as various nations strived to limit the effects of climate change and to reduce nuclear arsenals.

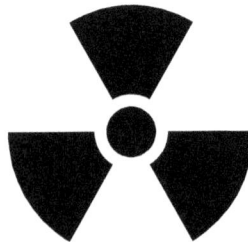

with the organization's perceived prospects of nuclear war. From the scientists' perspective, the lowest level of danger occurred during a four-year stretch from 1991 to 1995. During that period, they set the clock back to 17 minutes before midnight in the wake of the Strategic Arms Reduction Treaty between the United States and the Soviet Union.

Since 1995 for the most part the danger levels have steadily increased in the wake of tensions between India and Pakistan, a lack of progress in global disarmament, and North Korea's test of nuclear weapons as Iran expressed ambitions to obtain similar devices.

Since 1995, the only pullback of the clock away from the midnight doomsday hour came in January 2010 when scientists set the time back by just one minute as various nations strived to limit the effects of climate change and to reduce nuclear arsenals.

Chapter
3

Understand the Horrific Power of Nuclear Weapons

The nerve-wracking sensations of facing danger from nuclear weapons left countless people worldwide spellbound from the 1950s through the 1960s, in the wake of the U.S. bombings of Hiroshima and Nagasaki at the end of World War II. The massive waves of death and destruction emblazoned fear deep into the hearts of people across the globe throughout those generations.

The massive waves of death and destruction emblazoned fear deep into the hearts of people across the globe throughout those generations.

Largely because those tragic occurrences impacted people more than two generations ago, at least some of today's younger adults might lack any sense of urgency. For the most part, what little many of them might know about the subject comes from old film clips, movies and required classroom instruction during their school lessons.

At least from my view, the advent of the Internet, instant cell phone communications, and extremely violent video games have left many of our younger people numbed to the very real danger of widespread nuclear radiation that faces us all.

On the positive side, hopefully the recent catastrophic events in Japan and elsewhere will motivate people of all ages and from every culture to fully grasp the danger while also learning and implementing essential protective measures.

From the perspective of many people, just about every significant problem today seems to have an instant or relatively fast cure or solution. Quickie answers ranging from fast food to instant coffee and drive-thru windows might leave the impression in younger minds that "they will find a fix for whatever ails me" or for whatever problem that might come our way.

Sadly, though, this is not the case with weapons of mass destruction and particularly any destructive device or strategy designed to spread massive amounts of deadly radiation over an expansive area.

On the positive side, hopefully the recent catastrophic events in Japan and elsewhere will motivate people of all ages and from every culture to fully grasp the danger while also learning and implementing essential protective measures.

For this to happen with any degree of effectiveness on a widespread scale, people first need to grasp a comprehensive, snapshot-style understanding of the history of nuclear weapons, the various methods of such warfare, how such devices would be used to attack us, and ultimately the best methods of personal protection and of medical treatments.

James W. Forsythe, M.D., H.M.D.

Appreciate and Respect the Massive Power of Nuclear Weaponry

A single, normal-size nuclear bomb can destroy an entire city in an instant, killing hundreds of thousands or even millions of people within the blink of an eye—while also spreading massive amounts of deadly radiation across expansive areas for up to hundreds of miles.

"The discovery of nuclear reactions need not bring about the destruction of mankind any more than the discovery of matches."

-Albert Einstein

"The discovery of nuclear reactions need not bring about the destruction of mankind any more than the discovery of matches," said Albert Einstein, a 20th Century physicist and widely acclaimed genius who mastered the theory of relativity.

During the 1930s and 1940s, Einstein had encouraged U.S. President Franklin Delano Roosevelt to begin research and development of nuclear weaponry, largely because—as the scientist warned—our German enemies at the time had launched similar efforts.

Since the bombings of Hiroshima and Nagasaki at the end of World War II, the technology required to build and deploy nuclear bombs initially spread to the former Soviet Union and eventually to numerous other countries. Meantime, extensive improvements in communication techniques increased the danger that our enemies would learn specifics on how to implement this deadly technology.

The Japan
nuclear bombings
of more
than 66 years
ago marked the
only time that
nuclear bombs
have been used
in warfare.

"The world has achieved brilliance without wisdom, power without conscience," said the late U.S. Army General Omar Bradley, the first Chairman of the Joint Chiefs of Staff and the last-surviving commander to reach the rank of five-star general. "Ours is a world of nuclear giants and ethical infants."

The Japan nuclear bombings of more than 66 years ago marked the only time that nuclear bombs have been used in warfare. But since then, various nations and scientists worldwide have detonated nuclear devices more than 2,000 times.

As a practicing medical oncologist and a licensed homeopathic physician, for many years I have held the responsibility of treating numerous cancer patients impacted by radiation as a result of nuclear detonation experiments at the Nevada Test Site.

Avoid the Ravages of Radiation-Caused Cancers

Through the years, large numbers of patients from these deadly experiments actively tracked me down and asked that I implement the best-possible treatments to save their lives. As you might very well imagine, I felt a great degree of empathy for these patients, the victims of our reckless government and the deadly effects of radiation.

Now officially called the "National Security Site," the 1,360-square-mile expanse of desert in Nye County, Nevada, approximately 65 miles northwest of Las Vegas, began serving in 1951 as our government's designated site for exploding nuclear weapons.

Amazingly, for the first decade of these experiments our government was cold and careless enough to conduct these deadly procedures above ground. Failing to take necessary precautions, the scientists involved operated the facility in full disregard for public safety.

Failing to take necessary precautions, the scientists involved operated the facility in full disregard for public safety.

As a native of the Midwest born in 1938, I received my higher education and doctorate degree in California before serving as an officer and physician in the Vietnam War—before starting my medical oncology practice in the Northwest Nevada city of Reno in the early 1970s.

Within the first several years of starting my practice, steadily increasing numbers of people exposed to radiation from nuclear weapons testing began visiting my office for initial diagnosis and eventual treatment. Sadly, due largely to limitations from medical technology at the time, many of these patients eventually died of their radiation-caused cancers.

Imagine having to look someone in the eye and tell them: "Nothing can be done for you medically at this time. Our government has failed to protect you." If the truth be told, I would like to have said that our political and military leaders let our citizens down.

This extended period of time for symptoms to appear occurs when the person is exposed to radiation levels that are too low to cause sudden fatal ailments.

The Test Site Will Go Down in History as Shameful

Comprised primarily of mountainous and desert terrain, the test site location had been known as the "Nevada Proving Grounds" prior to the deadly experiments.

The many radiation victims that I treated were civilians who lived in desert communities outside of the primary nuclear blast zones. Nevada's mysterious and sometimes unpredictable high-desert winds blew nuclear fallout and the resulting radiation into various towns and small communities throughout Nevada, Idaho, Utah and Arizona.

As scientists had later discovered in the Japan communities surrounding Hiroshima and Nagasaki, cancer caused by radiation exposure sometimes takes many years or even decades to develop in an individual. This extended period of time for symptoms to appear occurs when the person is exposed to radiation levels that are too low to cause sudden fatal ailments.

Because of this factor, some aging people who were children or young adults when exposed to radiation from the Nevada tests are just now beginning to experience the symptoms of potentially deadly cancers.

In total, our government conducted 100 above-ground tests at the site. The first above-ground blast occurred when scientists dropped a 1-kiloton nuclear bomb on Jan. 27, 1951, at Frenchman Flat. The site's final above-ground test shot was "Little Feller 1" of Operation Sunbeam on July 17, 1962

Thus, anyone just now starting to experience the initial cancerous effects of nuclear radiation from the Nevada nuclear blasts is in his or her late 40s or older. Also, babies born in the initial years after the final tests faced the possibility of nuclear contamination. Scientists tell us that radiation can settle on farmland grasses eaten by milk-producing cows. Such milk sold in stores can pass the radiation on to children, who also faced danger from eating meat by products from animals.

Besides the Nevada experiments, scientists employed by the U.S. government also conducted 126 above-ground nuclear bomb tests outside of the continental United States—most of them in the Marshall Islands at the Pacific Proving Grounds. Through 1992, the government conducted 828 underground tests in Nevada.

"Our knowledge can only be finite, while our ignorance must necessarily be infinity," said Karl Popper, a 20th Century Austro-British philosopher and professor at the London School of Economics.

Testing Efforts Became Extensive

Researchers even placed mannequins near buildings or close to cars or inside of automobiles in efforts to measure the effects of blasts and of the resulting radiation.

The testing, and particularly the above-ground blasts, was far more extensive than many people realize today.

Determined to create near-realistic situations within the planned nuclear blast zones, scientists ordered the construction of numerous buildings. These structures were built using designs and materials specifications common in Europe and the United States.

Heightening the perceived intensity, many of these make-shift homes in ground-zero areas targeted for bombing and in nearby areas featured replicas of civil defense fortifications and even backyard shelters that some citizens were building at the time.

The efforts to document this destruction used the highest, most efficient technologies of the time. Crews installed high-speed movie cameras that generated images that many of us remain highly familiar with even today, such as paint actually melting on the side of walls. Researchers even placed mannequins near buildings or close to cars or inside of automobiles in efforts to measure the effects of blasts and of the resulting radiation.

"Our observation of nature must be diligent, our reflection profound, and our experiments exact," said Denis Diderot, a French writer, art critic and philosopher. "We rarely see these three means combined, and for this reason, creative geniuses are not common."

Sure enough, looking back these many decades following the Nevada experiments, it's relatively easy for many of us to serve as so-called "second-guessing Monday morning quarterbacks." Perhaps in the heat of the situation as the cold war intensified, scientists and governmental leaders were simply reacting in the best ways that they could possibly conceive at the time.

Even so, there can be little denying that these various experiments caused extensive physical suffering and persistent heartache among many innocent U.S. citizens.

Environmental Damage from the Testing Endangers the Public

Long after the bulk of the testing was completed, after the Nevada complex's nuclear bomb-blasting functions ended in 1992, officials determined that a whopping 300 million curies of radiation remained from those experiments.

Although many tests were conducted underground, some nuclear explosions occurred within thousands or even hundreds of feet of groundwater. Needless to say, by almost every account the site and perhaps surrounding areas remain one of the most

"As soon as there is life, there is danger."

-Ralph Waldo Emerson

radioactively contaminated regions in all of the United States and perhaps the world.

Ralph Waldo Emerson, the great 19th Century lecturer, philosopher, essayist and poet, told us so succinctly and eloquently that "as soon as there is life, there is danger."

Unquestionably our very existence involves risks of many kinds. Yet as citizens of the United States and of the world for that matter, each of us carries a responsibility to ourselves and to those who follow us to ensure that the world's physical environment remains safe and clean to clear the way for the abundance of life and to preserve nature's great potential.

The U.S. Energy Department maintains and operates at least 48 monitoring wells at the former test site. Researchers have found millions of picocuries of radiation of per liter of water under the blast zones. That's many hundreds of thousands of times greater than the federal standard of just 20 picocuries.

These results serve as an urgent reminder that extensive radiation exposure can endanger and obliterate life for extended periods, harmful levels that easily can last for many thousands of years.

Civil Litigation from the Nevada Bomb Blasts Spread

Bowing to political pressure and admitting that our government failed its citizens, in 1990 Congress passed the Radiation Exposure Compensation Act.

The legislation guaranteed $50,000 checks to each person who suffered cancer or other specified illnesses—or their surviving relatives, after living in specified areas of Nevada, Utah, Arizona or elsewhere in the American West. Claimants needed to live in certain counties between January 1951 and October 1958, or again from June 30, 1962, and July 31, 1962.

According to various published reports, the compensation sent to these people heralded as "downwinders" reached a combined $525 million by 2006. Of the total 13,500 claims filed, only 10,500 had been approved.

Of course, although such a check might seem an extremely large amount in the eyes of many, a mere $50,000 does not even come close to compensating for the pain, suffering and deaths caused by our government's reckless and arrogant procedures.

Still striving to "right this terrible wrong," in 2000 our Congress also passed the Energy Employees Occupational Illness Compensation Program Act. This legislation created medical benefits and

According to various published reports, the compensation sent to these people heralded as "downwinders" reached a combined $525 million by 2006.

71

compensation for those who suffered work-related illnesses during their employment within the nuclear weapons industry. The same legislation also allocated $100,000 compensation payments to those who transported ores, worked in mills or who mined uranium.

"An apology for the devil—it must be remembered that we have heard one side of the case," said Samuel Butler, an iconoclastic 19th Century Victorian novelist. "God has written all the books."

Our Government Thinks of You as Expendable

A compelling, unforgettable and must-read book by Carole Gallagher, "American Ground Zero— The Secret Nuclear War," published in 1993, gives irrefutable evidence that our government gave little concern about the lives of people downwind from the nuclear test blasts.

Following her research funded in part by the John D. and Catherine T. MacArthur Foundation, Gallagher quotes from a formerly classified, top-secret Atomic Energy Commission document that designated people who lived in the southern section of Utah as a "low-use segment of the population."

"I feel like we were really used, and I'll never trust our government again," Josephine Simkins of Enterprise, Utah, told Gallagher. From my perspective as a concerned physician, Simkins and the many others whose families were killed off or decimated by the radiation have every right to feel angry with our pitiless government.

Diligent and relentless in her pursuit for the truth and to reveal the atrocities inflicted by our government, Gallagher courageously revealed horrific details of a propaganda booklet that the U.S. Atomic Energy Commission had distributed to Utah residents. This deceitful, deadly and murderous propaganda advised them to "expect reports that 'Geiger counters were going crazy here today.' Reports like this may worry people unnecessarily. Don't let them bother you."

Like I say loudly and clearly, we should never fully trust everything that our government or any government says, particularly in matters of health and public safety. Today, the graveyards of isolated communities across Arizona, Utah, Nevada and Idaho are littered with the bodies and headstones of the countless people killed by our government's insensitive actions.

Packed with magnetic, compelling, unforgettable photographs, Gallagher's book quotes numerous former U.S. military personnel who were either forced to watch the nuclear blasts or who personally suffered extensive medical problems—in some cases as their offspring experienced similar extensive health difficulties.

"We had a post-flight briefing and the doctor said, 'Gentlemen, I've read your dosimeters. You've received half enough rems of radiation to kill you."

-Herbert Holmes

"The plane was crackin' and poppin,'" Herbert Holmes of Clarksburg, West Virginia, told Gallagher, when describing his harrowing experience at the test site as a U.S. military pilot in 1957 when he was 27 years old. "The explosion blew up about 4,000 feet, the shock wave hit and blows you another 2,000 feet. Straight up over a mile, this plane weighed well over 100 tons and it was like we were just a feather. We had a post-flight briefing and the doctor said, 'Gentlemen, I've read your dosimeters. You've received half enough rems of radiation to kill you.'"

Shockingly, our government also forced military personnel who filled trenches to witness the explosions, some able to see the bones of their own hands and fingers although their own eyes were closed during the height of the blasts. How many of them subsequently suffered from deadly cancers?

In the late 1970s, I wrote an article for the "Reno-Gazette Journal," then published as the "Reno Evening Gazette" and "Nevada State Journal," about cancer patients that suffered a high rate of the disease in Fallon, Nevada—often deadly illnesses generated by contamination exposure from the test site. I treated many of these patients. Some recovered and a number of them suffered painful early deaths.

James W. Forsythe, M.D., H.M.D.

Always Remain Skeptical When Scientists Say "It Can Never Happen"

As a highly trained physician taught to always follow established scientific criteria, I'm always skeptical whenever anyone—even other doctors—make casual but well-intended statements such as "it can never happen." To embrace and rely on such statements can emerge as a recipe for disaster.

Consider for instance the underground explosion of Dec. 18, 1970, at the Nevada Test Site, a test shot named "Baneberry" during an experiment entitled "Operation Emery."

Prior to the planned 10-killotonne nuclear bomb blast 900 feet below the earth's surface, based largely on previous experience scientists assumed that the experiment would contain all radiation underground.

To the apparent shock and dismay of some researchers, however, a huge cloud of radioactive gas spewed many hundreds of feet into the air shortly after the blast, which carried 6.7 megatons of radioactive material into a hot cloud that spread into California, Utah, Nevada, accross the U.S. to Canada, the Gulf of Mexico and the Atlantic Ocean.

This serves as a prime example of the urgent need for us all to take any statements such as "this is the way it always happens" with a certain degree of healthy cynicism.

75

This multiplied the concerns of highly experienced medical oncologists and homeopaths such as myself, since we have seen the resulting increased cancer rates of people who once had been assured that "nothing serious will happen."

Indeed, during the initial days following the March 2011 Japan nuclear disaster, much of the general public within that nation was advised never to worry. Concerned residents across that nation were told that the situation was well under control, and that any serious radioactive contamination of their communities and food and water sources was highly unlikely.

So, imagine the horror, fear, deep concern and worry that many of these people felt just eight days after the initial disaster when frustrated officials confirmed that signs of contamination had been found in that nation's food products in cow's milk and in groundwater.

This multiplied the concerns of highly experienced medical oncologists and homeopaths such as myself, since we have seen the resulting increased cancer rates of people who once had been assured that "nothing serious will happen."

Refrain From Panicking But Show Genuine Concern

Focused on the well-intended need to prevent panic, officials strived to assure the general public throughout the United States that American citizens on the West Coast faced no danger whatsoever from radiation released from several damaged nuclear power plants during the Japan crisis.

Exactly seven days after Japan's ravaging 9.0-magnitude earthquake and the killer tsunami,

James W. Forsythe, M.D., H.M.D.

monitoring stations in the California capital of Sacramento announced that radiation from the Japan disaster had already reached the Golden State.

When issuing the initial results of the oncoming radiation, officials were quick to assure the American public that the initial impact of this energy mass sweeping across the Pacific onto the U.S. West Coast was one-millionth of the range of danger levels.

A stream of scientists and physicists were interviewed on U.S. television throughout the weekend of March 19-20, 2011, virtually all of them telling viewers that Americans had nothing to worry about due to the miniscule levels of radioactive materials.

All along, skeptics such as I remained cognizant that whenever scientists tell us that "something can never happen," a possibility remains for unexpected and unwanted results such as the radioactive leak into the atmosphere after the 1970 nuclear test blast.

One widely known scientist even went so far as to tell national TV viewers that all of us in the United States born before the 1986 disaster at Chernobyl have miniscule levels of radiation in our bodies due to that Russian emergency.

Essentially, some researchers and public relations gurus seemed to be telling us 25 years after that

Now, imagine if you will a horrible dust storm that generated massive, high-speed winds in China several years ago.

event that we "have nothing to worry about concerning Japan, and you're just fine—aren't you—after Chernobyl? So, you should avoid any worries about what happened far away across the mighty and vast Pacific Ocean."

Massive Dust Clouds from China Have Covered the Western United States

To those who insist that nothing detrimental could ever happen to the American homeland as a result of the Japan disaster, I cite the occurrence of a mysterious and interesting weather event that happened several years ago.

My medical clinic in the Western United States is in Reno, Nevada, about 218 miles northeast of San Francisco, and 132 miles from Sacramento. Between Reno and those cities is the scenic Sierra range, where many mountain peaks hover well over 8,000 feet above sea level.

Putting this into additional perspective, please consider the fact that San Francisco on the U.S. Pacific Coast is 6,897 miles from Hong Kong on the other side of the Pacific at the eastern edge of China.

Now, imagine a horrible dust storm that generated massive, high-speed winds in China several years ago. For a period of several days beginning about one week after the China storm, a giant dust cloud hung over Reno—which sits at the eastern edge of the Sierra at the 4,500-foot elevation in the high desert of the Great Basin.

After this initially unexplainable and mysterious dust clogged the air, meteorologists announced that strong winds had blown this dirty air clear across the Pacific before pushing the airborne soil well into the Western United States, even past and over high-mountain areas.

For comparative reasons, specific pollutant levels from that event remain unavailable for in-depth analysis. Even so, I recall that several of my patients asked me during the time of the China dust cloud if they had reason for serious health concerns as a result. At the time, meteorologists assured the public to avoid any worries about public safety.

All these years later, in the immediate wake of the Japan nuclear power disaster, I could not help but wonder if the so-called experts might be wrong when they assured Americans that there should be absolutely no reason for worry or concern.

After all, since the China dust storm was able to send relatively thick, air-clogging pollutants clear around the world in such massive quantities, why should we have assumed that the Japan disaster would remain difficult-to-measure, miniscule levels of radiation from clear across the Pacific? Why should we have put our full faith into what our government and nuclear industry scientists tell us?

Even so, I recall that several of my patients asked me during the time of the China dust cloud if they had reason for serious health concerns as a result.

Always striving to push for the good health of all Americans, my level of concern increased one week after the Japan disaster.

Avoid Alarmist Reactions and Unwarranted Conclusions

Careful to avoid any hint of being an alarmist on this issue, and fully cognizant of the need to refrain from causing unnecessary panic, I began telling anyone who asked my opinion of the issue that: "I'm skeptical about what we're being told; I'm keeping an open mind."

Perhaps more than ever before, people from around the world and particularly some gullible Americans need to "question authority" in regard to such serious issues.

Always striving to push for the good health of all Americans, my level of concern increased one week after the Japan disaster. That morning, a highly respected doctor appeared on a morning news show to discuss the possibility of whether Americans faced potential danger from the Japan nuclear radiation leak.

Responding to an anchorwoman's queries, this expert essentially said that U.S. citizens within our homeland were absolutely not in any danger.

To prove his point, this analyst placed a few drops of greenish-blue dye into a small container filled with water. As expected, the water became filled with intense, difficult-to-see-through colors. Then, this commentator said that we should consider this as the concentration levels if the radioactive contaminants were confined to Japan.

Then, the analyst dropped a few additional dye droplets into a second water container of a much larger size than from the initial demonstration. This time as expected the overall coloring throughout the water in the second container appeared much lighter and easier to see through than the colors in the first container.

The resulting color in the second container, the commentator said, was an example of how dissipating the dye in a much larger glass was an example of how a substance is diluted and spread apart. He equated this to when a substance gets spread across a larger area than merely being confined to an original contamination zone.

And, finally, the commentator put the same amount of droplets into a third container, significantly larger than the first glass and much bigger than the second container as well. This time after he stirred the mixture the dye could hardly be noticed within the largest container. This, he said, represented what would happen if a dangerous substance is introduced into a much larger area such as the ocean.

Supposedly this demonstration was his way of showing that only highly dissipated levels of radiation possibly could get into the Pacific before spreading miniscule, harmless levels of these contaminants to the United States.

Always skeptical in such situations, as a highly trained physician familiar with industry-accepted

I have noticed that historically some meteorologists and scientists have been flat-out wrong when predicting the environmental impacts of sea and ocean currents.

testing procedures, I feel an urgent need to let the world know here that to the best of my knowledge such instances have never been tested in a scientific setting.

World Renowned Weather Events Signify That Scientists Can Be Wrong

Once again looking to historical events for potential answers or possibilities, I have noticed that historically some meteorologists and scientists have been flat-out wrong when predicting the environmental impacts of sea and ocean currents. Consider for instance the events that followed the tragic Deepwater Horizon oil spill in the Gulf of Mexico, beginning with an explosion that killed 11 men at an oil rig platform on April 20, 2010.

Just like in Japan where government and corporate officials failed to respond and take immediate and decisive action, following the Horizon accident our nation's politicians and executives at BP or British Petroleum waited too long to make vital decisions.

Now labeled as the petroleum industry's largest accidental spill, that disaster also showed that no matter how well-intentioned they might be, meteorologists and scientists can make significant errors in predicting the outcomes of environmental disasters.

As many people along the U.S. Gulf Coast know far too well by now, that tragedy's resulting oil spill caused far more environmental damage than some researchers had initially advised the public to expect.

Just like the tragic Japan disaster, officials found themselves responding to an emergency of a huge magnitude. All along, these responders and administrators had no previous real-life experience to use as a basis for the development and implementation of their strategies.

According to various news reports issued shortly after the Deepwater Horizon disaster began in the Gulf of Mexico, military responders and BP officials initially estimated that the broken sea-floor well was releasing oil at a rate of 1,000 barrels per day. By the middle of June just two months after the disaster began officials had increased those estimates to up to 60,000 barrels per day.

Compounding the problem, some observers began to question whether the oil spill area had expanded to a much broader zone than officials originally forecast. In the months that followed, various environmental organizations and wildlife preservation groups began to openly question whether BP had been forthcoming in releasing vital information.

With these lessons in mind, should the world trust statements issued by the Japan power company and by that nation's government? Should the public

By the middle of June just two months after the disaster began officials had increased those estimates to up to 60,000 barrels per day.

News reports revealed that from 1982 through 1984 more than 2,000 apartment units where constructed there, using radioactive steel that had been salvaged from a recycled nuclear power plant.

believe everything these authorities say about the issue? Or, is at least some degree of skepticism healthy?

Small-Scale Radioactivity Accidents or Oversights Occur

Accidents and human errors involving radiation on a much smaller scale have consistently and regularly plagued people across numerous societies since the 1950s.

The steadily increasing urgency of the need to respond to and address problems of radioactivity hits the news on a regular basis, although few people pay much attention.

One of the most heart-wrenching of these events occurred in 1982 in Taiwan, an island nation off the coast of mainland China. News reports revealed that from 1982 through 1984 more than 2,000 apartment units where constructed there, using radioactive steel that had been salvaged from a recycled nuclear power plant.

Human error, incompetence and sloppy government regulations contributed to many of the various radiation accidents or tragedies, exacerbated in 1983 when someone dismantled a discarded radiation therapy machine near Ciudad Juárez, Mexico. Authorities later determined that a truck used to transport the dismantled materials had sustained radiation contamination when coming in contact with materials from the deconstructed machine.

Meantime, the person who salvaged the radioactive device sold the metals for the eventual construction of other devices or tools such as legs for kitchen tables and restaurant tables—and for building material sent to the United States and Canada. Ironically, authorities finally discovered the problem when a radiation monitoring device at the Los Alamos National Laboratory detected excessive amounts of radioactivity from a truck that was delivering contaminated building materials.

Especially for those of us concerned enough to carefully monitor the dangers of radiation, this inspires an obvious and necessary question: "How much of the materials around us have been unintentionally radiated? Are similar dangerous materials making their way into the U.S. building supply chain? And, what if anything is being done to protect the general public from such occurrences?"

Among the many other incidents of accidental or malicious radiation contamination:

- **Brazil**: In 1987, scavengers dismantled a radiation-therapy machine that had been taken from a former medical clinic. These culprits sold the most dangerous parts of the machine, essentially as "glowing curiosities." According to news reports, at

Are similar dangerous materials making their way into the U.S. building supply chain? And, what if anything is being done to protect the general public from such occurrences?

In 1994 in the
community
of Commerce
Township, a
17-year-old boy
attempted to
construct a make-
shift, homemade
breeder nuclear
reactor in the
back yard of his
mother's home.

least four of the buyers died from radiation contamination and 250 other people suffered contamination.

- **Ukraine**: In 1989, at least six residents of an apartment building died and 17 others sustained excessive doses of radiation. Investigators discovered that the building's infrastructure contained a small capsule embossed in a concrete wall that held caesium-137, a highly radioactive material. Investigators determined that the capsule apparently had been lost in the 1970s, before being mixed with gravel eventually used for building construction.

- **Michigan**: In 1994 in the community of Commerce Township, a 17-year-old boy attempted to construct a make-shift, homemade breeder nuclear reactor in the back yard of his mother's home. According to various reports including a 2004 book by Ken Silverstein, "The Radioactive Boy Scout," the youth, David Hahn, had amassed radioactive materials by taking apart everything from clocks and smoke detectors to gun-sight devices. The various substances amassed by the boy reportedly emitted 1,000 times what scientists consider normal background radiation. Amazingly, in 1995, the U.S. Environmental Protection Agency designated the back yard as a Superfund Clean-up Site. Silverstein reported that authorities dismantled a back yard shed and burned it in Utah.

Such disturbing instances lead to still more questions, such as "How many other people including potential terrorists are dismantling various household objects to amass radioactive materials without being noticed?"

Sadly, there seems to be no comprehensive system to check such occurrence, marking another problem that signifies that each of us needs to remain diligent in our efforts to avoid the potential dangers of radiation.

"The enlightened ruler is heedful, and the good general full of caution," said Sun Tzu, a highly acclaimed Chinese military general from more than 500 years before Christ, and author of the still-widely-read "The Art of War." Perhaps more than ever, particularly in matters that involve radiation, officials in the United States and officials elsewhere must do much more to protect their citizens from such accidents.

After all, as the world's overall population swells while the coming decades and generations pass, wide varieties of radioactive devices are likely to get discarded—possibly endangering countless numbers of people.

"The enlightened ruler is heedful, and the good general full of caution,"

-Sun Tzu

Discover the Extreme Dangers Imposed by Radon

Designated by the symbol "Rn," radon actually is a chemical element that many of us first learned about while in high school chemistry class.

As a concerned medical oncologist always determined to warn the public of dangerous carcinogenic situations, I also feel motivated to issue an urgent warning here about the potentially extreme dangers of a substance called radon.

Perhaps many thousands or even hundreds of thousands of individuals nationwide are exposed to radioactive radon in their homes without even realizing they're endangered.

A tasteless, colorless and odorless gas, radon occurs due to the decay of uranium—the primary substance necessary in the construction of nuclear bombs. Designated by the symbol "Rn," radon actually is a chemical element that many of us first learned about while in high school chemistry class.

Considered one of the most common isotopes on Earth, uranium has a half life of at least 4.5 billion years—meaning the substance has an extremely slow break-down process. Since this isotope is relatively common, radon gas has been known to accumulate in many types of buildings and houses without occupants realizing that they face extreme danger as a result.

Researchers and experts in radon gas warn us that high concentrations of this chemical often build up in confined spaces such as attics and basements. People dedicated to maintaining good health sometimes find themselves startled to learn that high levels of radon emanate from spring water and even hot springs.

Through the past several decades, I have treated many patients for a variety of cancers that likely were caused by the radiation emitting from radon. Lots of these patients including those suffering from inoperable lung cancers first visited me far to late, long after the point where medical technology might have given them a fighting chance to survive.

Even so, like I often tell my patients, "Always walk away if a physician tells you that 'It's time to get your personal affairs in order, and your medical situation has passed the point of hope.'" Yes, thanks largely to integrative cancer treatments available through my clinic, at least some of these patients now enjoy good health after their cancers reverted to what many people in the general public refer to as "remission."

Many of these patients can be seen giving their heart-felt, true-life recovery stories in compelling online videos seen on my Website, DrForsythe. com. However, as I continue treating cancer patients from around the world I am saddened to realize that many cases of cancer from radiation and carcenogenic agents will be so astromomical that these patients will not be able to seek or have proper medical care.

Some doctors prescribe radon treatments for certain auto-immune conditions such as arthritis.

Check for Dangerous Radon at Your Home or Office

The increased urgency of the extreme dangers imposed by radon become clear when realizing that this chemical causes an estimated 21,000 cases of lung cancer yearly in the United States, making it the second leading cause of the disease behind cigarette smoking, according to a 2009 report by the Environmental Protection Agency.

A 2008 article distributed by the Lawrence Berkeley National Laboratory lists the highest concentrations of radon in the United States in Iowa and in southeastern Pennsylvania's Appalachian Mountain region.

Such contamination can occur in many areas of the country, and other nations also experience high radon levels such as County Cork, Ireland.

Compounding the problem and spreading the dangers, according to the same EPA report numerous homes have been built on landfills that contain uranium tailings.

Ironically, in the meantime, like many other potentially harmful substances such as opium poppies used in the production of morphine, radon has its own specific proven uses as a legitimate treatment of medical conditions. Some doctors prescribe radon treatments for certain auto-immune conditions such as arthritis.

Some medical professionals use radon to generate limited doses of low-grade radioactive water for certain treatments. Radon, in conjunction with various other materials such as items like seeds produced with gold or glass are administered for the treatment of certain types of cancer.

"Caution is the eldest child of wisdom,"

-Victor Hugo

Get a Radon-Testing Kit or Hire Professionals

Many hardware stores or home improvement supply stores offer relatively inexpensive kits designed for low-cost radon testing. Such easy-to-implement efforts can go a long way toward alleviating concerns, while also marking the first possible step toward decreasing the probability of radon-caused cancers.

"Caution is the eldest child of wisdom," said Victor Hugo, the 19th Century French author, poet and philosopher. To be sure, anyone who performs such an easy radon-checking test can make tremendous strides in generating safer conditions for themselves and for their loved ones.

Short-term radon testing kits used on the lowest livable level of a house take just two to seven days to complete. By comparison, long-term testing units can collect potential radon material levels during a period lasting up to one year. The experts stress that radon levels in a specific dwelling can vary

Ultimately, the primary method for reducing radon gas in a home is to us a "vent pipe system and fan, which pulls radon from beneath the house and vents it to the outside."

over time, due to certain fluctuating conditions such as weather factors.

With most store-bought devices, the user sends the test kit to the device's manufacturer for analysis. In addition, some radon-measuring devices work on open land before building construction starts.

For instances where tests detect excessive or potentially harmful levels of radon, the World Health Organization list several primary ways to revamp the structure. Among the primary potential measures:

- **Sump**: Install a sump system to pump the harmful gasses away from the structure.

- **Ventilation**: Install a "positive pressurization" ventilation system.

- **Depressurize**: Use a sub-slab depressurization system, essentially increasing ventilation under the floor.

- **Air flow**: Improve the overall air flow through the structure, improving ventilation.

Ultimately, the primary method for reducing radon gas in a home is to use a "vent pipe system and fan, which pulls radon from beneath the house and vents it to the outside," according to U.S. Environmental Protection Agency's "Citizens Guide to Radon."

Chapter
4

Discover the Basic, Essential Factors of Radiation

Before discovering the essential techniques for surviving nuclear tragedies, you need to know the basics of radiation. Understanding this phenomenon, how it occurs and its specific dangers serve as the basis for anyone determined to survive extremely harmful levels of such conditions.

In fact, many people fail to understand even the most mundane, basics of what radiation entails.

Since the advent of the first nuclear bomb blasts at Hiroshima and Nagasaki in August 1945, the concept of radiation has retained a mystic and almost surreal image from the view of many within the general public. In fact, many people fail to understand even the most mundane, basics of what radiation entails.

To the gullible general public, misconceptions and unfounded fears emerged during the 1950s and well into the 1960s. Many movie-goers during that era believed or at least worried about the concepts conveyed by the top science fiction films of the

Unseen except in unusual circumstances, radiation impacts each of us on a continual, almost non-stop hour-by-hour basis.

time. Perhaps the most famous movie storylines featured creatures such as aunts that grew to tremendous size when exposed to radiation.

The legendary 20th Century science writer Isaac Asimov once said that "individual science fiction stories might seem as trivial as ever to the blander critics and philosophers of today—but the core of science fiction, its essence has become crucial to our salvation if we are to be saved at all."

Sure enough, at least in the eyes of many observers, the world's most serious well-documented, real-life nuclear disasters seemed stranger than fiction. Even as events unfolded during the height of the Japan nuclear power disaster, for instance, some analysts already were applauding the heroics of the "Fukushima 50"—courageous nuclear plant workers who risked their lives in attempts to salvage the situation.

This seems even more admirable when we take into consideration the fact that for the most part under normal circumstances radiation is all around us in our everyday lives. Unseen except in unusual circumstances, radiation impacts each of us on a continual, almost non-stop hour-by-hour basis.

It isn't until radiation reaches extremely high dangerous levels that this often misunderstood phenomenon becomes a serious threat to human health. In worst-case scenarios, extremely high levels of radiation cause cancer, skin rashes and even death. The fact that such events are usually invisible to the human eye only seems to heighten the sense of mystery and even fear. This factor hails as a primary reason why rescuers who risk their own lives to eradicate radiation are sometimes perceived as "fighting an unseen monster."

From my view, such incomprehensible courage is almost impossible to put into adequate words, let alone to describe with any degree of accuracy. Indeed, as the famed legendary Renaissance period artist Leonardo da Vinci once eloquently stated, "the poet ranks far below the painter in the representation of visible things, and far below the musician in that of invisible things."

"The poet ranks far below the painter in the representation of visible things, and far below the musician in that of invisible things."

-Leonardo da Vinci

Although Invisible, Radiation Can Become Dangerous

Experts in physics tell us that radiation is actually comprised of energetic waves. In nature and throughout our everyday lives such energy travels through the space around us, and also through objects or mediums such as our bodies or other objects. For the most part, there are two basic types of radiation:

- **Non-iodizing**: For the most part, the specific atoms and molecules remain bonded to each other in pairs. As a result, the individual has no "floating"

95

Besides cancer, the many diseases or severe ailments often blamed on free radicals include life-ending or threatening events such as strokes and myocardial infractions.

or unbound characteristics that would increase the likelihood of certain types of cancer.

● **Iodizing**: This process generates free radicals, cancer-causing chemical reactions, created when electromagnetic waves—sometimes commonly referred to as "particles"—detach from the atoms or molecules that comprise basic substances. When a free radical develops, an extremely dangerous situation erupts because the atoms or electrons are no longer bonded in safe pairs. When allowed in the human body, free radicals—especially when administered at high levels—can cause severe cancers and even degenerative diseases such as severe skin damage, hair loss and organ failures.

Paradoxically, at least according to some medical experts, certain free radicals can emerge as beneficial to health—processes necessary to maintain life, such as the killing of potentially harmful bacteria.

However, excessively high levels of free radicals can seriously injure cells within the human body when roaming unattached atoms or electrons bond with otherwise healthy bonded pairs. Besides cancer, the many diseases or severe ailments often blamed on free radicals include life-ending or threatening events such as strokes and myocardial infractions.

Worsening matters, free radicals sometimes cause severe damage to the body's cellular DNA. In severe-case scenarios that involve extreme, extensive exposure to high levels of radiation over a prolonged period of time the body loses its natural ability to effectively replicate and create new cells.

To put this into clear perspective, think of these dangers this way: In healthy people, billions of cells naturally die off on a daily basis, and the body replaces them with healthy new cells. But the advent of excessive levels of free radicals causes damage to the body's internal DNA system, wrecking or destroying this vital process.

Some people exposed to excessive levels of radiation over prolonged periods develop cancer almost right away. Yet other individuals, particularly those exposed to lesser but still severe levels of radiation for limited periods, sometimes develop cancers several years or even decades after such exposures. For these individuals, the onset of such disease is delayed because their natural DNA's cell replication process was less severely damaged.

> Some people exposed to excessive levels of radiation over prolonged periods develop cancer almost right away.

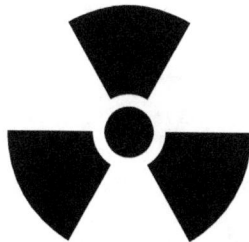

Chapter

5

Understand the Essential Basics of Nuclear Fallout

In order to increase your chances for survival after an unexpected nuclear bomb attack, you will need to know the basics entailed in the "nuclear fallout" process.

When a nuclear explosion occurs scientists refer to the spread of radioactive materials as "fallout" because such contaminants literally fall out of the resulting mushroom cloud or from the surrounding atmosphere immediately after the blast.

Hot particles litter the radioactive dust as winds and various atmospheric weather conditions spread radioactive contamination. While hot particles do not necessarily emit high temperatures when touched, they possess extensively high or "hot" levels of radiation. Scientists warn us that hot particles can emit from a variety of sources rather than just what most people commonly call the "ash" from fallout.

Scientists warn us that hot particles can emit from a variety of sources rather than just what most people commonly call the "ash" from fallout.

99

The contaminants might remain confined to a specified area, or the dangerous materials can spread over a much wider zone.

In fact, the hot particles process becomes increasingly complex, especially from the perspective of those of us who remain cognizant that the radioactivity can possibly—and is likely—to spread from one object to another as if a moving virus.

Besides from bombs in a nuclear fallout process, malfunctioning nuclear power facilities also can spread deadly hot particles following the breach of core reactors. Intensifying danger for workers at such facilities, hot particles also can sometimes be found outside nuclear reactors that remained undamaged, according to "Hot Particles at Dounreay," from a Nuclear Monitor.

As a form of radioactive contamination, hot particles can wreak havoc across the land and atop or inside the remnants of damaged buildings while also pushing radiation into the animal food chain—sparking a potentially deadly domino effect.

The Fallout from Radiation Reportedly Can Go "Global"

Apparently basing part of their conclusions on the various experiments at the Nevada Test Site, scientists also warn us that the spread of nuclear fallout can generate fairly unpredictable results. The contaminants might remain confined to a specified area, or the dangerous materials can spread over a much wider zone.

The potential spread of nuclear fallout to other regions hinges largely on the specific velocity and direction of winds during and after a blast, plus various other atmospheric conditions high above the earth.

Some combatants might choose to explode nuclear bombs above the ground, creating "air bursts" that are likely to spread radiation and damage over a much broader area than if the weapon were to blast on the ground.

The danger from a single nuclear blast can intensify on a widespread scale, perhaps even creating a worldwide phenomenon, when various fission and non-fission byproducts from the moment of the explosion become extremely small particulates. Intense, sun-like heat from a nuclear explosion's fireball can vaporize and eventually spread radioactivity.

Even today, intense argument and apparent disagreement flows among analysts and observers on the potential dangers to people many hundreds or even thousands of miles away from an above-ground nuclear blast zone.

As many people already know the term "ground zero" refers to the impact area of a bomb, particularly a nuclear explosion.

People at "Ground Zero" Face Certain Death

As many people already know the term "ground zero" refers to the impact area of a bomb, particularly a nuclear explosion. When a nuclear weapon blasts

So, remember this, "the further I am from ground zero, the greater my chances for survival."

on the ground, this term designates all points on land close to the detonation. And for an air burst the "ground zero" designation specifies the spot immediately below where the explosion occurs.

Also, in a much looser, less scientific sense some people might tend to designate the specific buildings where a nuclear reactor tragedy occurs as "ground zero." Although not used to describe any blast zone, such terminology might emerge for use as a point of reference to describe the degree of closeness to the most extreme danger point.

Of course, many of us think of the term "ground zero" as a reference to nuclear tragedies, but the phrase also is sometimes used to designate the specific point of an earthquake or other major disasters such as where a hurricane's eye hits land or where an epidemic first begins to spread into the population.

For anyone close to ground zero from a nuclear blast or from a nuclear reactor tragedy, the term is extremely important. So, remember this, "the further I am from ground zero, the greater my chances for survival."

The levels of radioactivity decrease the further away you are from ground zero. Lower levels of radioactivity mean the lesser chance or probability there is for deadly health impacts such as cancer, extensive skin damage and other severe health maladies.

Meantime, anyone unlucky enough to be at ground zero when a nuclear explosion hits is likely to get vaporized in an instant. Winds close to the blast zone will likely reach many hundreds of miles per hour, literally blasting almost every type of people-made object apart.

Some long-time residents of that region blame radioactive contamination of the food supply chain.

Beware of Food Supply Chain Contamination

As the people of Japan learned to their great regret following the nuclear reactor disasters, the spread of radiation can contaminate the food supply chain—a negative, potentially deadly impact that could possibly last for many generations.

Following the Chernobyl disaster for instance, according to various news reports, children born months or even years after the disaster suffered inordinately high levels of cancer. Some long-time residents of that region blame radioactive contamination of the food supply chain.

Cows and other animals many miles from the former Chernobyl nuclear plant ate from grasslands that had been contaminated with radioactive materials. These contaminates then were passed on to babies who were fed the milk or who ingested other animal by-products including meats. Even vegetables became a matter of suspicion.

The chances for survival increase for those who manage to eat only non-contaminated foods and water.

"You can be a king or a street sweeper, but everybody dances with the Grim Reaper," said Robert Alton Harris, a convicted murderer, when uttering his final words immediately before being executed in 1992 at California's gas chamber at San Quentin Prison.

Anyone who survives near a nuclear blast should avoid entertaining such doomsday, we're-all-going-to-die-anyway thoughts. If and when such an event should occur to you, no matter how dire ongoing conditions might seem at the moment, the chances for survival increase for those who manage to eat only non-contaminated foods and water.

Earth and Water Play Critical Roles

Primarily from a nuclear blast's ground zero and nearby areas, earth and water play critical roles in the spreading of radioactivity when those elements get vaporized.

Along with remnants from the explosion this process creates a deadly radioactive cloud. Such spectacular, eye-catching phenomena are depicted in vivid, haunting images such as those seen in photographs of the ill-advised U.S. nuclear tests from the 1960s and 1970s.

Commonly known as mushroom clouds due to their similarity in appearance to such plants, mushroom clouds are typically associated with nuclear explosions but also can emit from non-radioactive blasts caused by conventional weapons. The instability generated at ground level by a nuclear blast generates low-density and hot gasses in massive quantities, thus forming what scientists label as Rayleigh-Taylor instability.

This occurs when one fluid of lower density pushes against a different fluid of higher density. Researchers have known of this instability process for many years, since long before the first nuclear bomb blasts. As seen by telescope observations of other galaxies, gravity acts upon the fluids of different densities eventually leading to unstable disturbances.

Telescopic photos of the Crab Nebula, a constellation far from earth, reveal that "potential energy" can build up and eventually get released when such instability occurs. Using a term first coined by 19th Century Scottish engineer and physicist William John Macquorn Rankine, scientists warn us that this phenomena occurs when force fields or a specific configuration stores up energy within a specified position.

"Nothing in the world is more dangerous than a sincere ignorance and conscientious stupidity," said the Rev. Dr. Martin Luther King Jr., the legendary pacifist and civil rights activist. Indeed, when the subject comes to matters of mushroom clouds, those of us striving for the preservation

"Nothing in the world is more dangerous than a sincere ignorance and conscientious stupidity,"

-Rev. Dr. Martin Luther King Jr.

At Hiroshima, authorities estimate that about 70,000 people died instantly or soon after the blast, primarily from burns, vaporization, radiation and various related diseases.

of healthy life must remain diligent in perceiving such visions as extremely dangerous and deadly, rather than things of beauty and divine mystery.

Physicists know all too well that energy can never be destroyed. And therefore the unchangeable laws of nature dictate that mushroom clouds must move and disburse their energy elsewhere. Invariably this means such events can and will eventually move radiation to a variety of potential areas, ranging from a recontamination of ground zero to the ground and food systems elsewhere.

Learn Vital Lessons from Hiroshima, Nagasaki, Chernobyl and Elsewhere

While specific estimates of the total number of dead vary from the nuclear bomb blasts at Hiroshima and Nagasaki, various U.S. governmental reports indicate that many thousands of people died of radiation-induced cancers over a period of years following the blasts.

At Hiroshima, authorities estimate that about 70,000 people died instantly or soon after the blast, primarily from burns, vaporization, radiation and various related diseases, according to a U.S. Department of Energy report issued in 2010.

Based on a variety of estimates, officials believe that tens of thousands of other individuals who were near the Hiroshima blast zone died of radiation-caused illnesses—especially cancer—during the next five years through 1950. While accounts and estimates vary, there seems to be little doubt that many people who had been outside the blast zone, perhaps up to 100 miles away died of similar cancers in subsequent decades.

Today, those worried about potential radioactive fallout or contamination from nuclear reactor accidents should not be blamed for their concern about possible similar outcomes. According to a report by the Radiation Effects Research Foundation, numerous solid cancers and leukemia killed people within the Hiroshima region through 1990 at a rate above the expected statistical average.

"Cancer patients are lied to, not just because the disease is (or thought to be) a death sentence, but because it is felt to be obscene, in the original meaning of that word: Ill-omened, abominable, and repugnant to the senses," said Susan Sontag, a 20th Century intellectual, political activist and author.

While personally determined to tear down such misconceptions, as a medical oncologist and practitioner of homeopathy, I strongly urge anyone contaminated by radiation to refrain from giving up hope—especially if they have any chance of getting high-level, dedicated medical care. To those people, I say, "Please remember that today's medical technology has advanced to a far more effective level—now more than a half century after victims of the Hiroshima and Nagasaki blasts suffered immense physical pain and death."

According to a report by the Radiation Effects Research Foundation, numerous solid cancers and leukemia killed people within the Hiroshima region through 1990 at a rate above the expected statistical average.

Understand the Basic Physics Involved in Creating Mushroom Clouds

Partly for this reason, the detonations of nuclear devices far above ground never produce what we typically perceive as mushroom clouds.

When a nuclear explosion occurs the initial blast wave sends super-charged energy straight into the ground, before bouncing back straight up into the sky. The resulting energy essentially creates the effect of a hot air balloon, generating a cap bubble at the top in the form of a sphere similar in appearance to the top of a mushroom.

Eventually this rise of super-hot gasses reaches an equilibrium level, the point at which the cloud's height starts to equal certain temperatures of contaminated objects held by the deadly cloud structure. Partly for this reason, the detonations of nuclear devices far above ground never produce what we typically perceive as mushroom clouds.

Nonetheless, such blasts generate mushroom-shaped tops that lack all the various types of matter contained in clouds from ground-level nuclear explosions. Instead, the tops of clouds from above-ground blasts contain primarily particles that are highly radioactive.

"I have realized that the past and the future are all illusions, that they exist in the present which is what there is and all there is," said Alan Watts, a 20th Century interpreter, thinker and writer. Sure enough, unless you're fast asleep and in a dream, at any moment that you might see a mushroom cloud at a distance you should know enough to immediately begin to move as far away as possible from that object.

According to various scientific reports and publications, the eventual distribution of radioactivity by a mushroom cloud hinges on a variety of factors. Among them:

The existing or changing weather conditions play a huge factor in determining the direction and distance of a mushroom cloud's remnants.

- **Yield**: The bomb's level of explosive power. Obviously, smaller yields would likely result in the shortest, least destructive clouds while huge yields could lead to clouds extending upward for tens of thousands of feet.

- **Burst altitude**: The specific level of the blast, whether open-air or at ground level. This could impact the eventual height of the cloud, and ultimately the potential traveling distance of the various contaminants that it carries.

- **Weather**: The existing or changing weather conditions play a huge factor in determining the direction and distance of a mushroom cloud's remnants.

- **Terrain type**: The atmospheric movements of a mushroom cloud hinge largely on the immediate and surrounding terrain, such as conditions that normally cause prevailing winds to usually move

People exposed to extremely high levels of radiation usually die almost immediately or within a matter of days.

in a certain direction. Everything from ocean currents to mountain canyons might play an integral role in determining a mushroom cloud's movements.

- **Fission and fusion levels**: Nuclear fission occurs when an atom splits into smaller units. This happens due to nuclear reactions when two or more nuclei collide, thereby generating matter or products that differ from the object's original state.

If and when you're ever fleeing from what you perceive as a mushroom cloud that you think was generated by a low-yield explosion, your greatest concerns should focus on potential contaminants from the top or cap of the cloud, rather than from the stem. According to the "Nuclear Survival Manual" published in 2008, the mushroom clouds from such explosions carry 90 percent of the contaminants at the top and only 10 percent of deadly radiation within the stem.

Recognize the Dangers and Symptoms of Radiation Sickness

People exposed to extremely high levels of radiation invariably suffer from extremely severe health conditions that doctors list as "radiation sickness." People exposed to extremely high levels of radiation usually die almost immediately or within a matter of days.

James W. Forsythe, M.D., H.M.D.

Many victims who are exposed to a moderate or mid-level amount of radioactivity usually begin experiencing devastating symptoms starting within several days or weeks of the initial blast. Sadly, for many of these individuals, their cancers or related diseases will reach critical or fatal levels.

The third level encompasses people who are exposed to the lowest levels of radiation for limited periods. In some instances, these individuals do not begin experiencing the initial symptoms of cancer until many years or perhaps even several decades after their exposure to radiation.

This is among the primary reasons why in the wake of nuclear power plant disasters officials sometimes seek volunteers who are at least in their late 40s or 50s. Such efforts are not made because these people are considered "more expendable," but rather due to the fact they're more likely to eventually die of old age before cancerous symptoms start. Outcomes of this nature hinge largely on whether the volunteers are exposed to low or moderately low levels of radiation, rather than extremely high or undeniably deadly doses.

At the 1986 Chernobyl nuclear reactor disaster officials attributed the deaths of more than 50 nuclear power plant workers to the accident. Many of these brave individuals who fought admirably and bravely in an effort to lessen the damage died extremely painful radiation-caused deaths within a few weeks of their exposure.

111

That's not saying that people shouldn't keep trying to rebel against the facts of existence. Someday, who knows, we might conquer death, disease and war..

More recently in Japan, the 2011 volunteers hailed as the heroic "Fukushima 50" risked their lives in a desperate but well-focused effort to prevent widespread emissions of radioactivity from the damaged nuclear power generators and containment facilities. Like other people exposed to radiation, the ultimate medical outcomes of these brave and dedicated people will hinge on the levels of radiation, the total time of exposure and the effectiveness of any protective garments they wore.

"A hero is someone who rebels or seems to rebel against the facts of existence and to conquer them," said Jim Morrison, a 20th Century rock 'n' roll star and lead singer of the Doors. "Obviously, that can only work at moments. It can't be a lasting thing. That's not saying that people shouldn't keep trying to rebel against the facts of existence. Someday, who knows, we might conquer death, disease and war."

Respond Quickly to Symptoms of Radiation Sickness

Based on the outcomes of Hiroshima and Nagasaki, plus various nuclear accidents, doctors can say with much assurance that people who suffer from radiation experience a high probability of suffering from genetic damage, tumors and cancer.

People who suffer genetic damage caused by radiation exposure lack properly functioning genes;

the actual function of their cells' DNA process malfunctions. This in turn causes mutations in the cellular structures, generating organ damage, destroying certain immune functions, and damaging the body's ability to naturally create or replicate healthy new cells as current cells die off.

Amid the height of a nuclear disaster, the best ways to lessen the probability of radiation sickness is to:

- **Flee**: Get as far away as possible from the primary source of harmful, deadly radiation.

- **Time**: Spend as little time as possible in radioactively contaminated areas, in order to decrease the total amount of contaminates that the body absorbs.

- **Potassium Iodide**: Ingested in pill or droplet form under a variety of names, this inorganic compound can play a significant role in decreasing the body's exposure to readioactive iodine—thereby preventing or lessening the probability of thyroid cancer, perhaps the most prevalent disease caused by radiation.

In each of these primary strategies, you should strive to take immediate action in an effort to minimize potential radiation exposure and to prevent this harmful energy from immediately destroying your body's primary functions. Any attempt to wait for a period of time in order to ponder what to do next could prove fatal.

You also should avoid ingesting such medications when existing and ongoing radiation levels are only negligible with extremely small percentages of radioactivity.

Controversy Erupted Regarding Iodide Pills

Amid the first week after the Japanese nuclear reactor tragedy, arguments flared throughout the news media and in online chat rooms about the perceived need to ingest potassium iodide pills.

Across the United States, commentators, news anchors and scientists went on TV and radio, telling the public that Americans were silly or perhaps even foolish to even contemplate taking iodide pills as a protective measure from potential radioactive contamination from Japan.

To the contrary, however, at least from my professional opinion, "it's better to be safe than sorry." Certainly except in the face of extreme emergency conditions, you should only ingest an iodide pill under the direct supervision and recommendation of a certified health industry professional—preferably a doctor or more specifically a medical oncologist. You also should avoid ingesting such medications when existing and ongoing radiation levels are only negligible with extremely small percentages of radioactivity.

Once again, I feel motivated to tell people to use caution. All along, in preparing for a potential radiation disaster, you should always have such a pill readily available in case you should eventually face an urgent, emergency and need to take one. Even better, right now you should consider getting adequate supplies, enough for your entire family.

"Be like a Boy Scout—be prepared," I tell people. "You do not want to wait until it's too late to assist yourself and also to help those you love and need to protect."

Everyone also should realize there are certain potential health drawbacks when ingesting potassium iodide pills. First off, you should never consider such pills as a "cure-all" against the overall negative impacts of radiation poisoning. Largely because these pills contain far more of this substance than the bodily normally ingests, certain medical complications might result—particularly if these pills are taken by a single individual in overly excessive doses or quantities.

In order to sharply lessen their probability of getting thyroid cancer, people should take the pills shortly after any exposure to high radiation levels or immediately before they expect dangerous levels to hit. The pills are sold under a variety of name brands, including ThyroSafe® and Rising Sun Health®.

Complicating matters even further, as fears heightened across America of potential radioactive dangers from the Japan tragedy, the U.S. Food and Drug Administration issued a warning that fake iodide pills already were being sold via the Internet. Particularly across the U.S. West Coast, physicians and pharmacists in some communities reported that there had been a run on legally obtainable iodide pills.

Taking advantage of the panic among some consumers, price gouging ensued with some pills reportedly going as high as $15 a pop via the Internet—far more costly than when purchased under normal conditions.

On March 20, 2011, nine days after the Japan reactor tragedy, a sub-headline on a "Los Angeles Times" story on the issue stated: "One doctor's response to a patient's fear of radiation from Japan: For Americans the risk of exposure is close to zero, and pills can have harmful side effects."

To the contrary, while also mindful of the potential dangers imposed by potassium iodide pills, I advise patients never to trust the predictions of scientists and never to fully embrace and adhere to whatever government or corporate officials tell them about such issues. Instead, while careful to take the pills only in emergency situations, the need for advanced preparation should remain a top priority for consumers.

Sadly, as if to thumb their noses at the concerned general public in the United States, some mainstream news media outlets issued headlines implying that mindless, horrified Americans who sought such pills were displaying a "siege mentality." Taking advantage of the panic among some consumers, price gouging ensued with some pills reportedly going as high as $15 a pop via the Internet—far more costly than when purchased under normal conditions.

Various Other Types of Cancers Can Erupt

For patients, physicians and medical facilities various other challenges erupt after radiation

116

emergencies, because a wide variety of other cancer types also can emerge.

Compounding this problem, extensive scientific research since the 1940s has determined that radiation emits, produces or emerges from a variety of extremely dangerous elements. Each of these specific substances is likely to cause a specific type of cancer or other ailment. Among the primary concerns:

Each of these specific substances is likely to cause a specific type of cancer or other ailment.

- **Iodine-131**: This is the primary culprit that physicians and experts in radioactivity warn against, although these professionals also say the other elements also are likely to cause significant dangers of extreme concern. Iodine-131 robs the thyroid of its essential and necessary function, the production of critical hormones. When Iodine-131 is obsorbed by the body, a victim's thyroid gland can develop thyroid cancer. This is why potassium iodide pills can help pack the thyroid with iodine, thereby keeping radioactive iodine from entering this essential gland. Meantime, however, physicians warn us that these pills will not protect the body's other organs.

- **Cesium-137**: Capable of dissolving in groundwater, this nasty and vicious element can dart straight to the bones before developing cancers within that

Several of my other popular books that many cancer patients consider essential reading include "The Compassionate Oncologist."

section of the body and also leukemia that curtails or blocks the ability of bones to make essential red blood cells.

- **Strontium-90**: Although acting like calcium in strengthening or building teeth and bones, this sneaky culprit also can generate leukemia and bone cancer.

- **Plutonium-241**: When this element builds up in the bone or liver cancer can develop in those areas.

Needless to say, besides blast burns, extensive skin damage and disabled lung functions generated by the nuclear explosion, the various types of fast-emerging cancers can quickly end life or emerge into debilitating conditions that drag on for decades. Patients who get vital medical attention soon after symptoms emerge often increase their chances for survival. Thus, following a radiation episode, you always should watch out for early cancer signs such as lumps, weakness, extensive weight loss, pain, the degeneration of essential bodily functions, or other mysterious symptoms.

Several of my other popular books that many cancer patients consider essential reading include "The Compassionate Oncologist." There you will find in detail my findings that integrating non-traditional medicines with standard techniques often get far better results in treating cancers than simply administering highly dangerous chemotherapy and radiation treatments.

Geiger Counters Serve a Critical Role

As just about anyone who has watched scientific movies and fantasy films knows, Geiger counters play a critical role in detecting harmful levels of ionizing radiation.

Often easily available for purchase online or at a variety of stores, these portable, hand-held devices work non-stop when activated to detect gamma rays and beta particles emitted by ionizing radiation or nuclear radiation. For obvious reasons, these machines serve an essential function since these dangerous elements cannot be seen by the human eye during normal conditions.

From the movies and TV shows, viewers can see that scientists, geologists or explorers often use hand-held objects that look like microphones connected by a cord to the Geiger counter's primary machine. Many of the modern, palm-size units such as those shown in numerous TV news reports amid the Japan reactor crisis lacked the need for any microphone-style detector.

When the monitor detects radiation levels a clicking sound emits and a needle on a gauge or lamp moves toward higher numbers while conveying a condition that scientists call the "cascade effect." Each level of increased intensity indicates a higher, more dangerous level of radiation. Some Geiger counters are capable of detecting three

The other devices serve important functions for a variety of industries or services including the medical profession and for geological purposes such as finding uranium.

types of ionizing nuclear radiation; alpha, beta and gamma rays. The presence of such hazardous ionizing nuclear radiation can cause extrme health problems..

In 1908, German physicist Hans Geiger co-invented the device's original version with Ernest Rutherford. With help from one of his students, Walter Müeller, 20 years later in 1928 Geiger developed an improvement of the original device in order to increase the types of radiation that the machine could detect. Another scientist, Sydney H. Liebson, made additional changes in 1947 to make the device functional for a longer period.

Without question, you should consider Geiger counters as essential tools necessary to help ensure your survival during a radiation emergency. By detecting excessive, high levels of ionizing nuclear radiation— alpha, beta, and gamma rays— you will be able to locate extremely dangerous conditions and determine which areas to avoid.

In addition, many of the same stores or Websites that sell Geiger counters feature a variety of other types of machines that detect potentially harmful radiation levels. The other devices serve important functions for a variety of industries or services including the medical profession and for geological purposes such as finding uranium.

James W. Forsythe, M.D., H.M.D.

Emergency Responders and Industry Workers Use Shields

In an effort to protect themselves from radiation and its harmful effects, medical professionals, certain nuclear power industry workers and emergency responders use shielding devices or specialized protective clothing.

Extremely thick or heavily layered substances, particularly lead, in many high-density instances block or at least lessen the harmful energies especially gamma rays. Depending on circumstances or energy levels, such professionals use everything from aluminum and lead to concrete, soil and other objects.

Since you likely would lack protective clothing in such a medical emergency, if unable to flee the contamination zone, the best option might become to seek underground shelter.

When unable to put distance between yourself and the radiation and its primary source, do everything possible to shelter your body from this danger.

All along, remember that besides shelter and distance, your other ally is time. In most instances, the longer you wait within as much protective area as possible, the greater the probability that highly harmful levels of radiation will dissipate to less harmful levels.

In summary, scientists use a formula to calculate the levels of sievert exposure that are increasingly harmful over specified time periods at varying radiation intensities.

Understand the Basics of Harmful Radiation Levels

To the lay person, the many varying levels of potential radiation exposure might seem quite confusing and difficult to understand.

In order to make this learning process simple, just remember that everything hinges on the number or level of sievert that a person is exposed to over a limited or extended period of time. A sievert, designated by the symbol "Sv," specifies a unit of "dose equivalent" radiation. Scientists and doctors use this measurement to signify the level that radiation is absorbed into the body.

This measurement system also detects "gray" units that specify how much the radiation is absorbed into any material, and also a unit called the "weighing factor." In summary, scientists use a formula to calculate the levels of sievert exposure that are increasingly harmful over specified time periods at varying radiation intensities.

Everything comes down to how many sievert or millisivert a person is exposed to, and for how long. Low-level exposures during the immediate period of danger range from nausea, vomiting and diarrhea to headaches and fever.

Following a latent period during which no symptoms occur, patients exposed to more sievert than the body can handle suffer everything from fatigue, hemorrhaging and severe infections to shock and death.

The levels range from below 1 to 2 sievers at the lowest range, the least harmful levels of exposure. The danger at higher levels steadily intensifies, with each level of danger and increased severity hinged on the amount of time the person is exposed to a particular sievert level. The most severe level kicks into gear when the sievert level surpasses 30, the range of imminent or certain death.

Take Appropriate and Necessary Precautions

A compelling 2005 publication issued by the National Academy of Sciences serves an integral role in advising scientists, engineers and medical professions on the various types of cancers and exposures from radiation.

People at the sites of widespread radiation accidents and downwind from these mishaps face cancer of the bile duct, brain, breast, colon, esophagus, gall bladder, lung and liver. Other potential serious or fatal maladies or illnesses include leukemia and multiple myeloma, non-Hodgkins lymphomas, and cancers of various other organs.

"When radioactive elements decay, they produce energetic emissions that can cause chemical changes to tissues," the academy publication says.

Events that make such exposure possible include radioactive fallout from nuclear bombs.

"The average person in the United States receives a 'background' dose of about one-third of a rad per year. Different types of radioactive materials emit different types of radiation."

Among the specific types of radiation materials that you should be concerned with, during or after a radiation emergency:

Gamma rays or X-rays: Among the most deadly types of such materials, these can pass through your body—possibly after traveling long distances to reach you, before putting your internal organs in jeopardy. Events that make such exposure possible include radioactive fallout from nuclear bombs.

Beta radiation: The academy publication warns us that although this potentially deadly material travels "a few yards in the air and in sufficient quantities might cause skin damage; it can be a hazard if ingested or inhaled." The academy noted that within areas where residents received government settlements due to Nevada Test Site experiments or to individuals in the uranium milling, transportation and mining industries, drinking contaminated milk emerged as the primary source of beta-radiation exposure.

Alpha radiation: On the positive side, this material fails to penetrate the skin and the substance only travels an inch or two in the air. However, the academy says alpha radiation is "a hazard if ingested or inhaled." Thus, potential exposure to alpha radiation reigns as a concern for workers who transport, mine or mill uranium.

These various dangers mandate that all industries involved in the process take essential precautions to prevent employees from potential contamination.

Always Beware of Harmful Medical Tactics

Compounding the problem of potential dangers from radiation, overly cautious physicians sometimes expose patients to excessive and potentially cancerous levels of this dangerous material.

"Some medical professionals including allopathic physicians, dentists and chiropractors order far too many radiological procedures. I advise patients to take extreme caution when anyone recommends such tests."

Sadly, putting the health of their patients at great risk—in an effort to protect themselves from potentially frivolous lawsuits—some physicians and practitioners of various medical specialties order unnecessary tests involving radiation.

Although their efforts are well-intended, in the long run these medical professionals have caused much more harm than good to the health care industry and to patients as well.

"Some medical professionals including allopathic physicians, dentists and chiropractors order far too many radiological procedures, I advise patients to take extreme caution when anyone recommends such tests."

A predictable outcome emerged as a result, legislation that fails to impose significant tort reform or to cap unfounded, frivolous civil court claims.

"This has had a spiraling, detrimental impact on almost the entire medical industry," I warn any doctor or nurse who asks for my opinion on this issue. "Even in cases where a doctor or hospital wins as a defendant in court litigation that involves radioactivity, the court disputes have drastically increased the malpractice insurance premiums for physicians. This in turn has resulted in unnecessary costs that doctors must pay up to unmanageable levels."

Worsening matters from almost every perspective, generating a detrimental ripple effect some doctors have been forced to increase the fees that they charge patients. This necessary inflationary measure in turn forces medical insurance firms to push up the monthly premiums charged to consumers for health coverage.

As if pushing a dagger into the hearts of every dedicated physician and straight into the pocketbooks of innocent patients. Recently enacted federal legislation on insurance coverage does absolutely nothing to mitigate this problem.

When developing and eventually approving these detrimental, ineffective laws, inept, incompetent or ignorant politicians strived to put a lasso around an industry they know little or nothing about. A predictable outcome emerged as a result, legislation that fails to impose significant tort reform or to cap unfounded, frivolous civil court claims.

James W. Forsythe, M.D., H.M.D.

You Face Dangers as a Consumer and as a Citizen

These many detrimental factors endanger not only the health of consumers, but their finances as well. As if today's average citizen doesn't already have too much to worry about such as nuclear reactors, nuclear bombs and radon emitting from the earth, they're also being hit with financial problems ignited by our sue-happy society.

Various studies show that "the real problem is too much medical malpractice, not too much litigation," said Tom Baker in the "Medical Malpractice Myth," published in 2005 by the University of Chicago Press.

From my view, almost all medical sub-specialties share at least some of the guilt in generating this problem. Yet standard medical oncologists as an overall group seem particularly susceptible to over-ordering highly dangerous and often damaging medical testing procedures that involve radiation.

To put this into perspective, you might want to keep in mind that a standard single chest X-ray emits about one unit of radiation. By comparison, a standard CAT Scan or CT Scan of the chest or abdomen generates from 70 to 100 times more radiation. Sharply increasing the potential dangers even more, a PET Scan that uses nuclear

127

Consumers have a right to know of the extreme dangers involved, medicine imaging for medical testing has five times the radioactive dose of a CAT Scan or up to a whopping 500 times greater than a standard, lower-tech X-ray.

Undoubtedly, some practitioners within the nuclear medicine imaging industry are going to erupt in rage toward me, for even daring to point this out.

Consumers have a right to know of the extreme dangers involved. Although PET scan procedures are non-invasive, meaning they do not insert standard people-made objects into the body, this technique involves ionizing radiation—the same harmful materials generated by nuclear bombs and nuclear power reactors.

Who could blame patients for becoming highly concerned when they learn that many PET Scan procedures are done simultaneously or in conjunction with CAT Scan checks? A 2005 report in the "Journal of Nuclear Medicine" confirms that combined PET and CAT scans can subject a patient to up to 26 millisieverts, a range considered substantial.

Radiation from Accidents and Medical Tests Harms Vital Cells

Ionizing radiation from attacks and accidents put the body's vital and essential immune systems in great peril. Among specific bodily cells or regions of great concern:

- **B-cells**: In order for your body to survive and thrive at a biological level, B cells derived from bone marrow produce critical antibodies—essentially large Y-shaped proteins that target and locate potentially harmful objects that invade the body such as viruses and bacteria. Thanks largely to these amazing and essential defensive processes, healthy B cells can often adapt in their functions in order to ward off or block microscopic invaders.

- **T-cells**: Within the white-blood cell category, in a realm that scientists call lymphocytes, T cells play a vital and necessary role in maintaining your body's immunity. Healthy T cells have receptors necessary for recognizing and capturing antigens, which essentially are comprised of potentially harmful substances such as bacteria or pollen.

- **Natural Killer Cells**: Sometimes called NKCs or NK cells, they serve a major role in enabling your body to fight tumors or even to reject once-healthy cells that have been invaded by viruses. In order to kill or destroy these biological enemies that might otherwise lead to your own death, natural killer cells emit specialized

This leaves your body without the necessary weaponry to fight and protect you from its natural enemies that work on a microscopic scale.

proteins directly into an invading cell's plasma membrane. This forms a pore that destroys the invader.

To get a clear vision of how this process works in a healthy individual, think of the hit 1977 movie "Star Wars," the classic 1960s TV series "Star Trek," or almost any other sci-fi outer space movie where spaceships engage in intra-stellar battles. This ongoing fight of immunity happens with fairly similar tactics within your body, except on a microscopic scale rather than across an entire galaxy.

Just like in the movies, the B-cells, T-cells and "natural killer cells" that serve as your proverbial warships quickly identify and seek to blast away invaders. But these good guys that work non-stop to protect you under normal conditions can get obliterated or wiped out by even small doses of radiation. When this happens, your protective cells lose their vital fire-power. This leaves your body without the necessary weaponry to fight and protect you from its natural enemies that work on a microscopic scale.

Radiation's Negative Biological Effects Mirror AIDS

Radiation attacks and destroys your body's immune system in ways similar to the ravages of the often-fatal condition AIDS or "acquired immune deficiency syndrome." Like excessively high levels of radiation, AIDS obliterates essential B-cells, T-cells and natural killer cells while curtailing or blocking the creation of those necessary functions.

People suffering from AIDS, generated by Human Immunodeficiency Virus, gradually or suddenly lose their vital immune cells. This in turn produces a condition ripe for the development of cancers, even among young people who almost always would otherwise naturally ward off such disease.

Like AIDS, radiation destroys or severely damages an individual's ability to effectively fight off many types of microscopic invaders like viruses and bacteria. Invariably, for many victims of AIDS and radiation contaminations—which are not naturally related conditions—illnesses often progresses to a level that lay people call "incurable."

Thus, as a general rule, I tell my patients that if at all possible they should avoid being subjected to highly dangerous PET scan procedures, CAT scans or any X-rays that might be considered unnecessary.

Instead of using those procedures for diagnosis, I often recommend or at least suggest much less dangerous Nuclear Magnetic Resonance Imaging examinations that the public often refers to as "MRI scans." Another option entails the lesser-known process of infrared thermograph or "thermal imaging." Instead of using potentially dangerous levels of radiation emitted from machines, the thermograph processes employs natural, non-

I often recommend or at least suggest much less dangerous Nuclear Magnetic Resonance Imaging examinations that the public often refers to as "MRI scans."

Before agreeing to take any test or treatment that involves radiation, you should ask for detailed information on the amount of such materials and if other much less dangerous options are available.

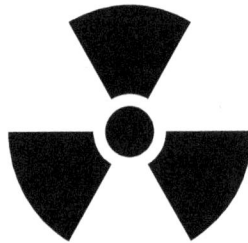

harmful levels of radiation that continually occur all around us amid usual conditions at room temperature. A breast thermogram is safer than a breast mammogram. The thermogram lacks any X-ray radiation and uses the heat radiating from the body to detect any physical abnormalities.

Before agreeing to take any test or treatment that involves radiation, you should ask for detailed information on the amount of such materials and if other much less dangerous options are available.

Chapter

6

Follow This Radiation Emergency Response Action Plan

Before and during a radiation emergency, you should take all of the following precautions in order to increase your probability of short- and long-term survival:

> Due to ongoing incompetence, selfishness and ignorance by such officials, you should never trust or assume the correctness of everything they say or advise.

- **Skepticism**: At all times, you should remain skeptical of what you're being told by government leaders and especially by representatives or lobbyists of corporations. Due to ongoing incompetence, selfishness and ignorance by such officials, you should never trust or assume the correctness of everything they say or advise. This holds true for you immediately after the onset of a radiation emergency, and during the initial weeks and months that follow.

- **Emergency kit**: Always keep handy an emergency kit available for immediate

133

In order to protect yourself from potential thyroid cancer if necessary, take along at least one potassium iodide pill—enough for you and for your entire family.

and necessary response to a catastrophic emergency including an earthquake, tsunami and particularly a radiation disaster.

- **Flashlight**: Keep a battery-powered flashlight in your emergency kit, plus enough batteries to last at least one week and preferably an entire month.

- **First-Aid Medical kit**: Within your emergency pack, keep a well-stocked medical kit that includes all the basic primary medical supplies.

- **Iodide pills**: In order to protect yourself from potential thyroid cancer if necessary, take along at least one potassium iodide pill—enough for you and for your entire family.

- **Radio**: Maintain and keep a functional battery-powered AM and FM radio, plus enough batteries to last an entire week and preferably a full month.

- **Water**: Pack the emergency kit with enough fresh water to last for at least an entire week, and preferably for longer periods.

●**Food**: Stock your emergency kit with enough compact, high-protein foods to last for at least one week at the very least for yourself and for your loved ones if necessary.

●**Clothing**: Take along enough fresh, clean, light-weight and functional clothing to last for a minimum of one full week.

●**Book**: A copy of the Emergency Handbook that you are reading now.

●**Geiger counter**: Without fail, be sure your emergency kit holds a functional Geiger counter and enough batteries to maintain its operations for an extended period. In the wake of a serious radiation disaster, you will need this device as an essential means of detecting or anticipating the worst danger zones.

In the wake of a serious radiation disaster, you will need this device as an essential means of detecting or anticipating the worst danger zones.

●**Duct tape and plastic coverings**: Keep your primary emergency kit or a secondary bag if necessary filled with ample amounts of duct tape and perhaps long stretches of plastic screenings for covering windows.

By planning ahead, you can avoid facing similar shortages in necessary supplies.

Like many medical emergency officials, I strongly advise you to take these advance precautions now, rather than waiting until later. This way beforehand you'll be positioned to take life-saving, immediate action at a moment's notice. Remember, in the wake of the Japanese nuclear tragedy, most store shelves in Tokyo more than 100 miles from the ground zero region consumers emptied store shelves of life's basic necessities. By planning ahead, you can avoid facing similar shortages in necessary supplies.

Prepare to Move Great Distances or to Stay in Place

Well before any potential disaster, you should keep in mind that everyone in your entire community—perhaps hundreds of thousands or even millions of people—likely will be in a state of panic if and when such an emergency occurs. As a result,well before and at the height of an emergency response, you should realize that the transportation system probably will be in a state of complete gridlock.

The lessons recently learned from the Japanese reactor tragedy should serve as a prime example of how transportation systems get clogged or damaged amid such extreme emergencies, and in the wake of such disasters. Coupled with six-hour lines at gasoline stations, damaged roads and clogged transportation routes drastically slowed emergency response efforts. Survivors from the damaged zones hundreds of miles north of Tokyo lost their abilities to escape in a quick and timely manner.

Worsening matters to the point of critical need, shelters for Japan's surviving quake and tsunami victims began running out of food and water just one week after the emergency began. Across the United States, particularly if a sizable radiation disaster occurs in more than one area, you should assume that our government likely will be slow to respond as well.

Highly familiar with the effectiveness and infrastructure of our overall U.S. medical industry, I fear that our government will lack the necessary medicines and supplies to respond fast in an effective and timely manner. From my perspective, amid the wake of such a disaster you should realize that the government will be ineffective. Although we're perceived as the richest and greatest superpower on earth, I worry that our nation lacks even the basic infrastructure necessary to respond to huge radioactive disasters.

Move Away from Highly Radioactive Zones

Making survival and long-term good health a top priority, you should strive to stay as far away as possible from ground zero. Remember, the highest and most deadly levels of radioactivity will likely be within that region.

Pay particular attention to the cracks at the sides and bottoms of doors, using the duct tape to fully block or minimize the amount of radiation that might seep into your shelter.

If you find yourself in an area that has a high or moderate level of radioactivity, but you are unable to travel to other areas, you should consider a survival technique called "shelter in place." This means staying in a single spot for an extended period. When forced into such conditions, first use your Geiger counter to determine the current radioactivity level.

If you determine that dangerous amounts of radiation are occurring, immediately use duct tape to place plastic wrappings securely on top of window and around doors. Pay particular attention to the cracks at the sides and bottoms of doors, using the duct tape to fully block or minimize the amount of radiation that might seep into your shelter.

People who discover that all buildings within the immediate area were destroyed by a nuclear blast should push together various items such as wood and aluminum to construct a short-term, makeshift shelter. Once you find shelter keep these factors among top priorities of your strategy:

- **Dissipation**: Particularly for people many miles away from ground zero, current radiation levels are likely to subside—usually within a matter of days, resulting in safer conditions.

- **Exposure**: For many survivors of the initial accident or attack, those exposed to lesser amounts of radiation will have the greatest chance of escaping cancer and related illnesses. When radiation levels are moderately low, you can go outside your shelter for limited periods of time without risking extensive contamination to your body.

- **Time**: Instead of worrying too much about time, you should make this your ally. The longer you are able to avoid continuous exposure to radiation, the greater your probability of maintaining good health or avoiding disease.

Besides the many lessons to learn and activities to enjoy, always prepare to get the most out of your experiences while seeking the fulfillment of your personal dreams.

"Mistakes are a fact of life. It is the response to the error that counts," says Nikki Giovanni, an African-American poet born in 1943.

Enjoy Life to the Fullest

Until such time as any major disasters such as radiation tragedies, feel free to enjoy life to the fullest.

Besides seizing the many lessons to learn and activities to enjoy, always prepare to get the most out of your experiences while seeking the fulfillment of your personal dreams.

To do anything less would be a disservice to us, to our families and even to our countries.

All along, those of us mindful of our world's many potential major emergencies should always remain prepared to take decisive action to save ourselves without hesitation. To do anything less would be a disservice to us, to our families and even to our countries. And, although I help champion the need to remain skeptical of our country's government, like many other patriotic Americans I remain loyal to our country and to the banner of freedom that many others worldwide covet and strive to generate for their own nations.

As the future generations pass through the continual march of time, let us all work together while continually mindful of the need to keep our earth, air and water as clean and as contamination-free as possible.

We, our children, our grandchildren and subsequent future generations depend on the tough decisions and actions that we make today. While considering myself as a public servant and a dedicated physician striving to treat patients from around the globe, I promise to strive to the best of my abilities to lessen the suffering and to eradicate the illnesses that people from many cultures might suffer— particularly from the ravages of nuclear radiation.

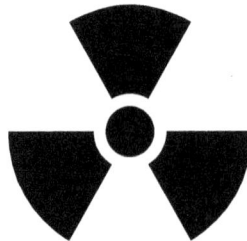

About the Authors

James W. Forsythe, M.D., H.M.D., is an author, anti-aging physician, and integrative medical oncologist specializing in the use of human growth hormone to combat the symptoms of aging. A native of Detroit, Michigan, Forsythe has won widespread acclaim for his many medical achievements in the battles against cancer. Details on Dr. Forsythe's medical practice and on his numerous books can be found at his Website, DrForsythe.com

Wayne Rollan Melton: A former editor-on-loan to "USA Today" in Washington, D.C., he has served as an entertainment columnist, society columnist, senior business writer, government reporter and a crime reporter specializing in major tragedies. Melton is the founder of the "Emergency Handbooks" series. For details on Melton's various books, visit EmergencyHandbooks.com